T0195477

Illustrated

DICTIONARY OF
MIDWIFERY

THIRD EDITION

Illustrated

DICTIONARY OF MIDWIFERY

—— THIRD EDITION ——

Joanne Gray, Rachel Smith and Caroline Homer

ELSEVIER

ELSEVIER

Elsevier Australia. ACN 001 002 357
(a division of Reed International Books Australia Pty Ltd)
Tower 1, 475 Victoria Avenue, Chatswood, NSW 2067

Copyright © 2022 Elsevier Australia. 2nd edition © 2018 Elsevier Australia.

1st edition © 2009 Elsevier Australia: this edition was published under licence from Elsevier Limited

First published in 2005, Illustrated Dictionary of Midwifery, Winson, McDonald © 2005 Elsevier Limited, UK. All rights reserved

ISBN: 978-0-7295-4399-6

Notice

Practitioners and researchers must always rely on their own experience and knowledge in evaluating and using any information, methods, compounds or experiments described herein. Because of rapid advances in the medical sciences, in particular, independent verification of diagnoses and drug dosages should be made. To the fullest extent of the law, no responsibility is assumed by Elsevier, authors, editors or contributors for any injury and/or damage to persons or property as a matter of products liability, negligence or otherwise, or from any use or operation of any methods, products, instructions, or ideas contained in the material herein.

National Library of Australia Cataloguing-in-Publication Data

A catalogue record for this book is available from the National Library of Australia

---

Content Strategist: Libby Houston
Content Project Manager: Fariha Nadeem
Copy edited by Leanne Peters
Cover by Georgette Hall
Typeset by GW Tech
Printed in China

Last digit is the print number: 9 8 7 6 5 4 3 2 1

Contents

About the authors

Joanne Gray, PhD, RM
Professor of Midwifery
Centre for Midwifery, Child and Family Health
Faculty of Health
University of Technology Sydney
New South Wales, Australia

Rachel Smith, MMid(Hons), RM
Midwifery Education Consultant
Maternal, Child and Adolescent Health
Burnet Institute
Victoria, Australia
Adjunct Fellow
Centre for Midwifery, Child and Family Health
Faculty of Health
University of Technology Sydney
New South Wales, Australia

Caroline Homer, PhD, RM
Co-Program Director
Maternal, Child and Adolescent Health
Burnet Institute
Victoria, Australia
Emeritus Professor of Midwifery
Centre for Midwifery, Child and Family Health
Faculty of Health
University of Technology Sydney
New South Wales, Australia

Preface

It has been more than a decade since the publication of the Australian and New Zealand edition of the *Illustrated Dictionary of Midwifery*, and there have been important global advances within the profession of midwifery. With the publication of the State of the World's Midwifery (SoWMy) reports (2011, 2014 and 2021), The Lancet's series on midwifery in 2014 and the most recent analysis of the impact of midwives in 2020, the focus on the difference high-quality midwifery care can make became truly global. These groundbreaking publications shifted the focus on midwifery from what has been a local or national approach to a more international agenda. Midwives are increasingly recognised as the key provider of sexual, reproductive, maternal and newborn healthcare in all countries. In recent years, however, significant challenges have been identified including social, professional and economic issues and the impact of gender inequities. In 2020, the COVID-19 pandemic further impacted the ability of midwives to provide woman centred care and highlighted the importance of universal health coverage and the provision of essential services to all women and newborns.

The International Confederation of Midwives (ICM) provides global leadership and also supports country-level midwifery associations to drive changes in practice, regulation and education. The ICM provides international direction with important documents such as the *International Definition of the Midwife*, the *Essential Competencies for Midwifery Practice*, *Global Standards for Midwifery Education* and the *Global Standards for Midwifery Regulation*. With the development of standards and policy documents, it is important to have accepted definitions such as those found in the *Illustrated Dictionary of Midwifery*.

While this Dictionary has been edited with midwifery students in mind, midwives may find it a useful resource in their everyday practice. The Dictionary uses woman-centred language and is based on the most recent evidence. A number of diagrams are also included to aid understanding of key terms.

We hope you enjoy this resource and find it useful in your practice.

Joanne Gray
Rachel Smith
Caroline Homer

University of Technology Sydney, Australia

Note from the Authors

The authors recognise that individuals have diverse gender identities. Terms such as pregnant person, childbearing people and parent can be used to avoid gendering birth, and those who give birth, as feminine. However, because women are also marginalised and oppressed in most places around the world, we have continued to use the terms woman, mother or maternity. When we use these words, it is not meant to exclude those who give birth and do not identify as women.

Aa

abdomen the enclosed area beneath the diaphragm and above the pelvis containing the organs of digestion and the liver. The rectus muscle of the abdomen covers the anterior wall and is capable of great distension to accommodate the gravid uterus and distended bladder.

abdominal relating to the abdomen, e.g. *abdominal pregnancy* where the embryo develops in the abdominal cavity.

abdominal adhesion the binding together by abnormal fibrous bands of normally separate internal structures/organs, sometimes causing pain and loss of movement. May occur following caesarean section or other surgical procedure.

abdominal breathing excessive movement of the abdominal wall during respiration; often seen in neonates with immature lungs. Can be indicative of respiratory distress.

abdominal cavity the space between the diaphragm and the pelvic cavity lined by the peritoneum and containing the liver, gall bladder, intestines, stomach and spleen. The kidneys are situated on the posterior abdominal wall and behind the peritoneum.

abdominal examination assessment of the abdomen using three senses: observation, palpation and auscultation; this is usually done during pregnancy to assess growth of the fetus and to determine its position, lie and presentation.

abdominal girth measurement of the abdominal circumference.

abdominal pain severe regional discomfort which inhibits normal activities causing the sufferer to seek midwifery or medical attention.

abdominal palpation the part of the abdominal examination in which the operator feels the abdomen to detect resistance, or absence of resistance, indicating the size and position of internal contents.

abdominal pregnancy (SYNONYM ectopic) occurs whereby instead of embedding within the reproductive system, the embryo embeds itself outside the uterus and starts to grow on the intestinal wall within the abdomen.

abdominal regions the division of the abdomen into named sectors in a three-by-three pattern (*see* Fig. 1).

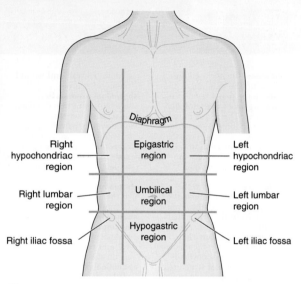

Figure 1
Abdominal regions

abduction the movement of individual parts of the body away from the midline.

abnormality a deviation from the usual or what is normal; a condition not found in the majority of individuals.

ABO adverse birth outcome.

ABO blood grouping the genetically determined classification of human blood as determined by the presence or absence of antigens.

ABO incompatibility (haemolytic disease of the newborn, also known as HDN or erythroblastosis fetalis) this can occur where the maternal blood group is O, containing both anti-A and anti-B antibodies, and the fetus is of group A, group B or group AB. Transplacental crossing of maternal antibodies may lead to haemolysis of fetal erythrocytes in various degrees of severity,

ABO incompatibility		
Group	Erythrocyte antigen (agglutinogen)	Serum antibody (agglutinin)
O	A and B absent	Anti-A and anti-B
A	A present	Anti-B present
B	B present	Anti-A present
AB	A and B present	No antibody present

causing severe jaundice in the early newborn period.

aboriginal having existed in a region from the beginning. For example, *Australian Aboriginal and Torres Strait Islander peoples* relates to the Indigenous peoples of Australia and should be spelt with a capital A when used.

abort premature ending of a pregnancy, usually before 20 weeks' gestation.

abortifacient a drug or other substance which may intentionally or inadvertently induce an abortion.

abortion the induced termination of a pregnancy before the age of viability.

abrachia congenital absence of arms.

abrasion superficial injury to tissue, usually as a result of trauma.

abruptio placentae the separation of part or all of a normally situated placenta prior to birth which results in bleeding. The bleeding may be visible vaginally but all or some may also be concealed within the uterus (*see* Fig. 2).

abruption a tearing away.

abscess a local collection of pus. Abscess formation is not uncommon in the breast following acute mastitis. Other common sites are in the Bartholin's glands at the entrance to the vagina and in the pouch of Douglas.

absorb to soak up fluids or gases. Components are drawn into one another across a membrane, becoming a unified whole.

absorbable surgical suture material used to close an incision or wound which does not require removal.

absorption the ability of the body to engulf matter, fluids or gases into the circulatory system.

abstinence to go without; avoidance of or refraining from, e.g. alcohol.

abuse cruelty or mistreatment of one person by another. Can be verbal, emotional and/or physical.

acardia absence of a heart. This congenital condition is rarely seen now except in conjoined twins as it can be detected by ultrasound scan

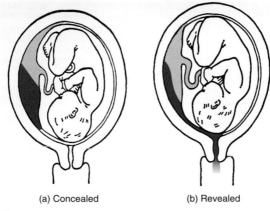

(a) Concealed   (b) Revealed

Figure 2
Abruptio placentae (a) concealed (b) revealed

and termination of pregnancy offered.

acardius acephalus absence of heart, head and upper parts of the body.

accelerate *see* augment.

acceleration phase (SYNONYM active phase) period of labour in which the greatest cervical dilation is achieved, commonly defined as between 4 and 10 cm.

accessory additional or supplementary, e.g. abdominal muscles are accessories to respiration and to pushing in the active second stage of labour.

accessory lobe of the placenta (SYNONYM succenturiate placenta) placental tissue supplementary to the main organ and connected to it by blood vessels.

accoucheur a professionally educated person who attends women in childbirth; usually a midwife or doctor with obstetric training.

accountability to answer for one's conduct; the requirement that a professional person accepts responsibility for and explains their independently performed actions upon request.

accreditation the acknowledgment of prior qualification/competence to perform or provide a skill or set of skills.

accreta complete attachment, as in *placenta accreta*, where the placenta invades and is inseparable from the uterine wall.

accretion adhesion of parts that are normally separate.

acephaly congenital absence of the head.

acetabulum a hemispherical depression situated on the lateral surface of the innominate bone (sides of the pelvis) into which fits the head of the femur (thigh bone).

acetone a chemical compound which is the simplest form of ketones.

acetylcholine a molecule that is important as a neurotransmitter. It is particularly important in the stimulation of muscle tissue.

achondrogenesis a type of short stature in which the person's limbs and trunk are shorter than usual.

achondroplasia a genetically acquired disorder, where growth of the long bones is affected resulting in short stature. The person's head often appears larger, the trunk is of normal size and intellect is normal.

achromatic lacking in colour. Red blood cells may lack colour in certain types of anaemia.

acid–base balance the state of equilibrium existing in the body when the body fluids achieve their appropriate pH value, e.g. blood pH 7.4, gastric juices pH 2.3, urine pH 4–5.

acid-fast bacillus classification of bacteria by their ability to hold an administered dye when its removal is attempted with acid.

acidaemia an accumulation of acid in the blood altering its predominantly alkaline state.

acidity degree of sharpness or sourness of taste; hydrogen ions are freely given out when dissolved in water.

acidity of the stomach relates to the acid–alkaline climate of the stomach.

acidosis a state created by depletion of the body's alkaline reserve and disturbance of the acid–base balance. Results from the body metabolising fat for energy instead of carbohydrate.

acinus (PLURAL acini) a small hollow sac or lobule lined by secreting cells and containing a duct.

acme peak, height; most painful part of a uterine contraction.

acne inflammation or sepsis in small sebaceous glands in the skin; commonly occurring on the face, chest and back.

acne neonatorum small white spots seen on an infant's skin.

acquired not inherited, developed in response to intentional or environmental exposure.

acquired immune deficiency syndrome (AIDS) progressive disease caused by the human immunodeficiency virus (HIV) which reduces the body's response to infection and tumour formation. Death occurs due to generalised debility and an opportunistic infection or tumour. HIV can be passed to the fetus/baby during pregnancy or breastfeeding.

acquired immunity enhanced resistance of a host to disease by passive or active exposure stimulating antibodies to develop.

acrocyanosis a reduction in the amount of oxygen delivered to the extremities. Common and considered normal in newborn babies due to immature circulation.

acromegaly a hormonal disorder that results from too much growth hormone (GH) in the body. The name 'acromegaly' comes from the Greek words for extremities ('acro') and great ('megaly'). The facial bones can also be affected.

acromial referring to the acromion.

acromion the triangular bony extension of the scapula which forms the point of the shoulder.

ACTH see adrenocorticotrophic hormone.

actinism the ability of ultraviolet (UV) radiation to cause chemical changes in the skin. This occurs when jaundiced neonates are exposed to UV light; the bile pigment in the skin is broken down.

active birth a term coined by Janet Balaskas who founded the active birth movement. Women are encouraged to be active during labour.

active first stage of labour period of time where the woman experiences regular painful uterine contractions, a substantial degree of cervical effacement and more rapid cervical dilatation from 5 cm until full dilatation.

active immunity resistance to disease resulting from exposure by infection or vaccination.

active management of labour a process of intervention intended to prevent and/or manage prolonged labour. It includes rupturing the membranes and augmenting labour with oxytocin.

active management of the third stage of labour an oxytocic drug is administered at the birth of the baby, the cord is clamped and cut soon after and controlled cord traction is applied to deliver the placenta. Also known as AMTSL.

acupuncture traditional Chinese therapy in which fine needles are inserted along specific lines or meridians in the body.

acupuncture point the point on the meridian at which the acupuncture needle is inserted.

acute describes a condition having a rapid onset, with pronounced symptoms but short duration.

acute abdomen name given to any condition which causes acute pain and tenderness over the abdomen.

acute circulatory failure where the cardiovascular system cannot meet the tissue needs for gaseous, nutritive and other substances. The failure may be caused by low blood pressure due to haemorrhage, loss of tension in the arteries or slow heartbeat.

acute fatty liver disease a complication of pregnancy, in which there is fatty necrosis, atrophy and destruction of the liver. Jaundice and itching are usually the initial symptoms.

acute inversion of the uterus a turning inside out of the uterus. An acute obstetric emergency of the third stage of labour.

acute nephritis inflammation of the nephrons caused by infection, allergy or loss of blood supply. Characterised by proteinuria and haematuria.

acute renal failure occurs when the person's kidneys do not function effectively leading to an inability to secrete urine and maintain normal homeostasis. Can be due to inadequate blood flow or severe infection and is a severe adverse effect of pre-eclampsia.

adactylia congenital absence of fingers or toes.

adaptation the ability to adjust in structure, form or function.

addiction a craving for, or loss of function without, the presence of the substance to which the body has become habituated.

additive a substance added to another to create a specific characteristic; a drug or chemical which may be added to another drug, intravenous infusion or food and administered at the same time.

adduction the movement of body parts towards each other or the midline of the body.

adherent placenta a placenta that does not separate from the myometrium during the third stage of labour. Surgical removal can be performed; *see* placenta accreta, placenta increta, placenta percreta.

adhesion abnormal fibrous joining together of normally separate body parts or organs including parts of the intestines following caesarean section.

adipose tissue connective tissue containing fat cells and fibrous areolar bands.

admission the procedure or right of entry; process followed in registering a person for care in hospital.

adnexa adjoining or accessory organs or tissues; the uterine adnexa are the ovaries and fallopian tubes.

adnexal relating to adnexa.

adolescence the period between puberty and adulthood; the teenage years.

adoption a legal process by which the biological parent relinquishes parental responsibility for a child and non-biological parents acquire all rights and responsibilities.

adrenal glands two endocrine glands which are situated on the upper poles of the kidneys, the hormones of which regulate fluid and electrolyte balance, metabolic rate and the 'fight or flight' system.

adrenaline (US: epinephrine) one of the hormones secreted by the medulla of the adrenal gland.

adrenocorticotrophic hormone (ACTH) hormone secreted by the anterior lobe of the pituitary gland, its target being the adrenal cortex where it stimulates the production of corticosteroids.

advanced embryo selection a preimplantation genetic test that enables the selection and transfer of embryos that are likely to have normal chromosomes.

advanced maternal age considered to be women over 35 years of age pregnant or giving birth.

adverse event unintended or unintentional harm or suffering arising from any aspect of healthcare management.

adverse reaction severe, life-threatening response to the administration of, for example, a drug, the opposite or contrary effect not occurring in the majority of people receiving similar treatment.

advocacy to act or intercede on behalf of another and in the best interest of another person.

aer- prefix meaning air or oxygen gas.

aerobe an organism requiring oxygen for maintenance of life.

aerobic requiring air or free oxygen for metabolism and life.

aerobic exercise exercise done to increase the work of the heart and metabolism in order to maintain fitness.

aetiology the study of factors related to the causes and origins of disease such as lifestyle, genetics and social conditions.

afebrile absence of fever.

affective concerned with or arousing feelings or emotions; emotional.

afferent carrying towards the centre, e.g. nerves towards the spinal column, blood vessels to the heart.

afibrinogenaemia loss of fibrin from the blood; occurs in association with disseminated intravascular coagulation (DIC), a complication of severe hypertension in pregnancy or catastrophic haemorrhage.

AFP see alpha-fetoprotein.

afterbirth the colloquial name given to the placenta and membranes expelled from the uterus after the birth of the baby.

aftercoming head the head following the birth of the body in a breech birth.

afterpains painful contractions of the uterus occurring after birth and commonly felt by multigravid women in the early puerperium and especially during breastfeeding.

agalactia a lack of breast milk.

age of consent statutory age at which one may give permission for medical treatment and voluntary participation in sexual intercourse. This varies in different jurisdictions across the world.

agenesis absence of an organ.

agenitalism a body without recognisable sex organs.

agglutination a process of clumping or coalescence.

agglutinin an antibody found in serum which, when added to an antigen on the surface of the erythrocyte, results in agglutination of cells.

agglutinogen an antigen which when injected into the body stimulates the formation of agglutinin and causes agglutination.

agnathocephaly a congenital abnormality in which there is a small chin, displaced mouth and approximate fusion of the eyes, which are low set.

agranulocyte a leucocyte (white blood cell) which, unlike a monocyte or a lymphocyte, does not contain granules.

AIDS *see* acquired immune deficiency syndrome.

air the mixture of atmospheric gases surrounding the earth containing approximately 21% oxygen and 79% other gases and capable of sustaining respiration.

air embolism air that is present in the vascular system or heart causing an obstruction to blood flow. This is abnormal and can be fatal.

air hunger a type of deep sighing respiration caused by imbalance of gases in the blood stimulating the respiratory centre.

air passages all the spaces through which air passes— nares, nasal cavity, pharynx, mouth, larynx, trachea and bronchial tree—on its way towards the lungs.

airborne infections transmission of pathogenic organisms on droplets of moisture in the air from one person to another without direct contact.

airway any of the devices used to maintain patency of the respiratory passages and prevent obstruction, used during anaesthesia and recovery.

ala wing-like processes or projection usually of bone, e.g. *ala of the sacrum*.

alba white substance, e.g. *lochia alba* (*see* lochia).

albicans white, e.g. *Candida albicans*.

albinism hereditary condition in which there is a lack of the pigment melanin in the skin such that the skin, hair and eyes are devoid of colour. The condition may also be associated with visual problems.

albumin a protein substance which is the main constituent of animal tissues. Serum albumin found in the blood is essential for carrying bilirubin.

albuminuria the presence of albumin in the urine.

alcohol (SYNONYM ETOH— ethanol) a fluid containing inflammable, intoxicating spirits which alters the cerebral function and consciousness.

aldosterone hormone secreted by the adrenal cortex which has diuretic properties.

alignment organs or tissues are in optimal position to one another, e.g. when an episiotomy is repaired the edges must be in alignment to ensure future comfort and function.

alimentary pertaining to food or nutrition, as in *alimentary tract*—the whole digestive canal from mouth to anus.

alkalaemia a change in the pH level of the blood from 7.4 to a slightly alkaline pH which will be detrimental to health.

alkali a compound which reacts with acids to form salts.

alkalinity the quality of being alkaline, containing more hydroxyl than hydrogen ions. Fluids can be measured on the acid–base balance (pH) on a scale of 0 to 14, strong alkalines being 14 and strong acids 1. Water, being mid-scale and neutral, has a pH of 7 and blood a pH of 7.4.

alkaloids organic nitrogenous compounds, many of which are of medicinal value.

alkalosis an abnormal condition where the pH of body fluids is > 7.45 as a result of too much alkaline hydroxyl (bicarbonates) and not enough acid (hydrogen).

allantois a membranous sac that develops from the posterior part of the alimentary canal and is important in the formation of the umbilical cord and placenta.

allergen a substance to which an individual has an abnormal response, such as itching skin, swelling, redness of the skin and mucous membranes including the eyelids.

allergic, allergy, allergic reaction a hypersensitivity reaction resulting from exposure to an allergen which may be a common substance in the environment such as pollen, feathers, etc. If the response is very severe, anaphylactic shock may occur, a condition which is life-threatening.

alpha-adrenergic mechanism autonomic nerve pathway mechanism through which excitatory responses occur as a result of the release of adrenergic substances such as adrenaline and noradrenaline.

alpha-fetoprotein (AFP) a byproduct of fetal protein metabolism identifiable in maternal serum and amniotic fluid. Quantitative assessment can be used as the basis of an antenatal screening test for the detection of fetal abnormality, especially spina bifida, Down syndrome and twin pregnancy. Further diagnostic tests are indicated.

alveolus small hollow cavity (i.e. air pocket) in the lungs where oxygen is exchanged for carbon dioxide; the milk-secreting structures in the breasts.

amastia failure of development of secondary sex characteristics and congenital absence of breast tissue.

ambient surrounding, as in *ambient temperature*.

ambulatory walking.

ambulatory care care not requiring an overnight stay in hospital.

amelia congenital absence of the extremity of one or more limbs.

amenorrhoea absence of the monthly menstrual bleed. This includes the period before menarche and women after the menopause. It is usually a term reserved for those of reproductive age and is a characteristic feature of pregnancy, certain diseases (e.g. anorexia nervosa) or severe emotional trauma.

amino acids a large group of organic compounds found in the blood; derived from protein in the diet and essential for building and repair of cells.

amitosis simple cell reproduction in which there is division of the nucleus and cytoplasm.

ammonia alkaline gas formed by the decomposition of proteins, amino acids and other nitrogen-containing substances.

amnesia inability to remember experiences; loss of memory. May be due to trauma, emotions or artificially induced, so that the woman who is lightly anaesthetised during caesarean section does not recall the procedure.

Amnihook (SYNONYM amniohook or amnicot) an instrument that can be used to artificially rupture the fetal membranes and allow amniotic fluid to drain.

amniocentesis an invasive procedure in which a needle is inserted through the abdominal wall and uterus into the amniotic sac and liquor amnii. Fluid containing fetal cells is withdrawn (*see* Fig. 3). Fetal cells obtained are cultured for chromosomal abnormalities and karyotyping as one method of prenatal diagnosis. There is a small risk of miscarriage occurring following this procedure.

amnioinfusion procedure to replace fluid which has drained off when membranes have ruptured prematurely and there is a risk of cord compression. Physiologically normal saline at body temperature is introduced into the amniotic cavity.

amnion the inner of the two fetoplacental membranes containing the amniotic fluid (liquor amnii).

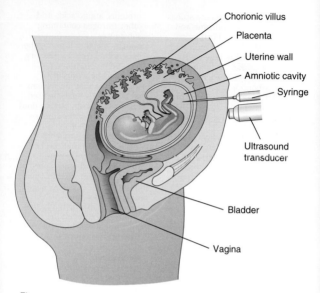

Figure 3
Amniocentesis

amnionitis inflammation of the amniotic membrane. This is usually due to infection.

amnioscopy introduction of a fibre optic instrument into the uterus to visualise the fetus.

amniotic cavity the space in the uterus occupied by the fetus, placenta and amniotic fluid, and lined by the amniotic membrane (*see* Fig. 4).

amniotic fluid (SYNONYM liquor amnii) the almost colourless fluid surrounding the embryo and fetus in intrauterine life, thought to be formed by secretion from the amniotic membranes and fetal urine.

amniotic fluid embolism entry of liquor amnii into the maternal circulatory system. A rare and serious condition leading to shock and maternal collapse which can be fatal.

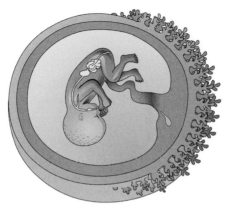

Figure 4
Amniotic cavity

amniotic sac the membranes within which the fetus develops.

amniotomy the procedure of artificially rupturing the fetal or amniotic membranes (*see* Fig. 5). Sometimes undertaken for observation of the liquor amnii as a means of assessment of the fetal condition, for the induction of labour, or to augment the first stage of labour. There are risks associated with this procedure.

ampulla the dilated end of a tube; the end of the fallopian tube furthest away from the uterus.

ampullary tubal pregnancy a conceptus which implants in

the distal end of the fallopian tube rather than the uterus (*see* Fig. 6).

AMTSL active management of the third stage of labour.

anadidymus conjoined twins joined at the pelvis or lower.

anaemia lack of red blood cells, a low haemoglobin concentration or haematocrit on examination of the blood.

anaemia of pregnancy may be a true anaemia or may be a reduced haemoglobin due to haemodilution—termed physiological anaemia.

anaerobe a microorganism not requiring oxygen to sustain growth.

anaerobic infection infection caused by organisms which

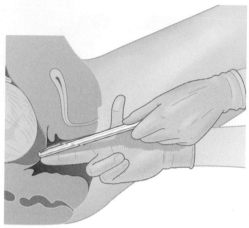

Figure 5
Amniotomy

do not need oxygen in order to multiply.

anaesthesia loss of consciousness induced by drugs usually administered prior to a surgical procedure.

anaesthetic agent used for inducing anaesthesia.

anaesthetist a doctor who specialises in the care of the anaesthetised patient.

anal (COMBINING FORM ano-) pertaining to the anus, as in *anal incontinence, anoplasty.*

anal incontinence involuntary leakage of faeces due to defective functioning of the anal sphincter which closes the rectum.

anal orifice the opening into the rectum.

anal verge the margins or edges of the sphincter which closes the rectum. Can be damaged in childbirth.

analgesia an agent used to render a person or area of tissue insensitive to pain without loss of consciousness.

analgesic drug used to produce analgesia.

analysis the breakdown of fluids or concepts, including research, into their component parts.

anaphylactic reaction, anaphylactic shock a collapsed state induced by

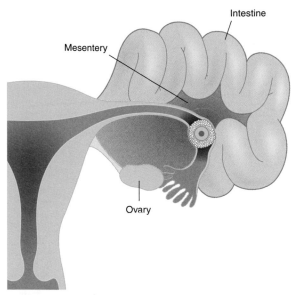

Figure 6
Ampullary tubal pregnancy

hypersensitivity to an antigen; the term applied to the respiratory distress and circulatory collapse that may be caused by drugs, snake venom, bee sting, a vaccine or certain foods.

anaphylaxis a severe allergic reaction. Soft tissues swell up and the airways can become obstructed making the condition fatal. An injection of adrenaline (epinephrine) is often given in an attempt to reverse this process.

anastomosis the creating of an opening between two cavities, tubes or organs. It may occur spontaneously or be accidentally or deliberately created during a surgical procedure.

anatomy the branch of science relating to the relationship between different tissues and organs of the body.

ancillary staff, ancillary services, ancillary support a person, service or support provided in addition to central activities.

andro- prefix meaning man or masculine.

androgen a hormone believed responsible for promoting male secondary sex characteristics and function.

android pertaining to the male gender.

android pelvis description of the deeper, more conical shape of pelvis seen in some women which can cause labour to be prolonged or sometimes obstructed.

androsterone an androgenic steroid found in male urine.

anecdotal information based on observation or an account from one person.

anencephalia the bones forming the vault of the skull and the cerebral hemispheres and cerebellum of the fetus are absent. A congenital condition that is not compatible with extrauterine life.

anencephalus a fetus with signs of partial or complete anencephalia.

aneuploid having an uneven number of chromosomes.

angina pectoris a condition that is often just called angina. It is characterised by chest pain due to ischaemia (a lack of blood and hence oxygen supply) of the heart muscle.

angiogram an X-ray image of a blood vessel into which dye

has been injected. May be performed postnatally if a deep vein thrombosis is suspected.

angioma a tumour composed of vessels—haemangioma (blood) or lymphangioma (lymphatic).

angiotensin a protein which causes vasoconstriction thereby raising the blood pressure.

angle of inclination of the pelvis the angle formed by the horizontal plane of the pelvis with the anteroposterior diameter of the pelvic inlet.

ankyloglossia a congenital abnormality in which the frenulum of the tongue is shortened prohibiting movement and speech; tongue tie.

ankylosis joint stiffness or immobility due to disease, trauma, surgery or abnormal bone fusion.

annual practising certificate allows a midwife to practise in a particular country. Usually issued by the regulatory authority or the government.

anococcygeal referring to the anus and coccyx, and the muscles between them.

anococcygeal body a mass of muscular and fibrous tissue situated between the anal canal and the coccyx.

anode a positive electrode to which negative ions are attracted.

anomaly a deviation from the normal.

anoplasty an operation performed to refashion the anus. Sometimes offered after a fourth-degree tear.

anorchia the absence of one or both testicles.

anorexia nervosa an eating disorder of psychological origin characterised by aversion to food; predominantly affects teenagers and results in emaciation and amenorrhoea.

anorgasmy (anorgasmia) failure to experience orgasm.

anovular unassociated with ovulation.

anovular menstruation menstruation not associated with the prior release of an ovum.

anoxaemia low level of oxygen in the blood; associated with asphyxia.

anoxia a state without oxygen; asphyxia.

antacid a pharmacological preparation used for neutralising acid in the stomach.

antagonise to neutralise the effect of a substance.

antagonist a drug that neutralises or counteracts the effect of another.

ante- prefix denoting before or preceding.

anteflexion bending forward. Used to describe the position of the uterine fundus in relation to the cervix and vagina.

antenatal (SYNONYM prenatal) occurring before birth; during pregnancy.

antenatal care the provision of care during pregnancy to provide support, information and observations and to detect and investigate risk factors and deviations from normal in the wellbeing of the mother and development of the fetus.

antenatal haemorrhage/ antepartum haemorrhage (APH) bleeding during pregnancy from the 20th week of gestation; indicates a deviation from normal, e.g. placenta praevia, abruptio placentae, cervical infection or erosion.

antepartum before birth.

anterior situated before or to the front, referring to the forward part of an organ.

anterior fontanelle the fibromembranous area on the head of the fetus or neonate situated between the frontal, sagittal and coronal sutures.

anterior–posterior diameter of pelvic outlet the distance between the middle of the symphysis pubis and the upper edge of the third sacral vertebra.

anteroposterior from front to back.

anteroposterior vaginal repair surgical procedure in which the upper and lower walls of the vagina are refashioned to reduce problems caused by overstretching and damage during the second stage of labour.

anteversion, anteverted inclined or tilted forward. The uterus is normally anteverted.

anti-sperm antibodies can develop in men or women and interrupt or adversely affect the movement or function of sperm leading to problems with fertility.

anthropoid ape-like, as in *anthropoid pelvis*.

anthropoid pelvis ape-like in character, the anteroposterior diameter is much greater than the transverse diameter. There is more space posteriorly than anteriorly so occipitoposterior positions of the fetus are more likely.

anthropology the study of people and their development, e.g. over time (*evolutionary anthropology*) and in relation to culture or rituals (*cultural anthropology*).

anti- prefix meaning against or preventing.

antibacterial preventing the growth of bacteria, usually a fluid or lotion.

antibiotic an antibacterial preparation or medicine offered when bacterial infection is present.

antibiotic resistance organisms not affected by antibiotics; symptoms of infection continue.

antibodies (immunoglobulins) a class of substances formed by the body in response to an antigen.

antibody titre the strength or quantity of antibodies present. These are measured in a series and comparisons of the levels made; the level measured may indicate recent or past exposure to an antigen. If levels are rising this indicates that the body is currently fighting antigens or infection.

anticoagulant a substance which prevents or restricts clot formation.

anticonvulsant a therapeutic agent which prevents or stops convulsions.

anti-D gamma globulin *see* Rh immune globulin.

antidepressants drugs used in the treatment of depression.

antidiuretic hormone the secretion of the adrenal gland which prevents excretion of urine, thereby controlling water loss from the body.

antidote an agent used to counteract the effect of poison or a drug.

antiemetic drug given orally or by injection to prevent or treat nausea and vomiting.

antifungal a drug or cream which prevents growths of fungi. During pregnancy *Candida albicans* in the vagina is not uncommon; it may be treated with antifungal cream or pessaries.

antigalactic a drug which suppresses the formation of milk in the mammary glands.

antigen a substance that brings about production of antibodies as an immunologic response.

anthelmintics agents used to eradicate intestinal worms (helminths) from the body. In endemic areas, a preventive anthelminthic treatment is recommended for pregnant women after the first trimester as part of worm infection reduction programs.

antihistamines a group of drugs used to block or diminish production of histamine which is released following tissue damage. Used in the treatment of various allergic conditions, e.g. hay fever.

antihypertensive a drug which lowers blood pressure.

antimicrobial a drug which prevents the growth of microscopic organisms.

antipruritic a drug, lotion or cream which is effective in the treatment of itching.

antipyretic a drug given to reduce a high body temperature and alleviate the symptoms of fever.

antiseptic a lotion which discourages the growth of microorganisms.

antiserum any serum obtained from human or animal blood which contains naturally derived antibody properties as a response to exposure to a specific disease. This can be injected into another person with the aim of protecting them from the disease, e.g. tetanus.

antispasmodic relieving or preventing spasm of smooth or striped (striated) muscle.

antithrombin substances in the bloodstream that may affect coagulation by inactivating thrombin.

antithrombolytic stocking applied to the legs to enhance the circulation thereby reducing the risk of deep vein thrombosis. Routinely applied before caesarean section in some maternity units.

antitoxin an antibody prepared from blood or plasma of an infected person or animal and introduced into another to counteract the toxin causing damage to the body.

anuresis retention of urine in the bladder.

anuria no urine is being formed.

anus the terminal end of the digestive tract.

aorta the large arching artery arising from the left ventricle of the heart.

aortocaval compression (*see also* vena cava) inability of the vena cava to return blood to the heart and the aorta to pump it to the lower limbs due to restricted lumen caused by the weight of the pregnant uterus (*see* Fig. 7). Occurs when the woman is lying on her back in the third trimester of pregnancy.

apareunia inability to perform sexual intercourse for physiological or psychological reasons.

aperient laxative or purgative which will cause bowels to move, relieving constipation.

Apert's syndrome a rare disorder that includes craniosynostosis, craniofacial anomalies and severe symmetrical syndactyly (cutaneous and bony fusion) of the hands and feet. It is autosomal dominant.

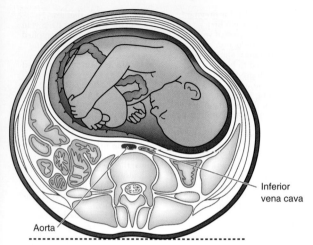

Figure 7
Aortocaval compression

Inferior
vena cava

Aorta

Apgar score a quantitative
scoring mechanism developed
by Dr Virginia Apgar, used for
determining the condition of
the infant within 1, 5 and
10 minutes of birth. It
assesses five features with a
maximum score of 2 being
assigned to each: heart rate;
respiratory effort; muscle
tone; response to stimuli
(reflex irritability); colour.

aphtha small white spot or
small ulceration on mucous
membrane that can be caused
by the fungus *Candida
albicans*.

aphthous vulvitis Infestation
of the vulva with
thrush.

aplastic incomplete or
defective structural
development.

apnoea the absence or
cessation of respiration; no
breathing movement.

**apnoea alarm mattress, apnoea
monitor** a machine which
records breathing and sounds
an alarm if breathing stops. A
small pad on which a baby
lies and which sounds an
alarm if the baby stops
breathing.

The Apgar scoring system (to assess neonatal condition at birth)			
Score			
Sign	0	1	2
Heart rate	Absent	Slow—below 100	Fast—above 100
Respiratory effort	Absent	Slow, irregular	Good, crying
Muscle tone	Limp	Some flexion of the extremities	Active
Reflex irritability	No response	Grimace	Crying, cough
Colour	Blue, pale	Body pink, extremities blue	Completely pink

aponeurosis a white, flattened or ribbon-like tendinous expansion, usually serving to connect a muscle with the parts that it moves.

apoplexy sudden impairment of neurological function, especially that resulting from a cerebral haemorrhage; a stroke.

appendicitis inflammation of the vermiform appendix. Uncommon in pregnancy though dangerous as pregnant women do not display the classic symptoms.

appendix vermiformis a wormlike diverticulum of the caecum, varying in length from 7 to 15 cm, and measuring about 1 cm in diameter.

applicator hollow rod used to introduce a soft structure (e.g. a tampon) or medicine (e.g. pessary) into a part of the body which cannot easily be reached.

appropriate for gestational age (AGA) describes a fetus or newborn baby whose size is within the normal range for the gestational age.

approximate to situate next to each other; to bring two tissue surfaces together, as in the repair of a tear or episiotomy.

apyrexia no fever present.

aqua (LATIN) water.

aqueous solution a water-based fluid which may carry other substances dissolved in it.

arachnoid the web-like delicate middle meningeal membranes covering the brain and spinal cord.

arcing spring contraceptive device a diaphragm introduced into the vagina to act as a barrier to sperm penetration.

arcuate ligament the ligament stretching across the subpubic arch of the pelvis.

arcus tendineus a thickening, generally known as the 'white line' in the pelvic fascia, which gives origin to part of the levator ani.

areola the coloured or pigmented area surrounding the nipple, which extends in pregnancy; usually, as much of the areola needs to be in the baby's mouth for successful breastfeeding.

areolitis inflammation of the areola around the nipple as a result of cracked nipples and poor feeding position.

arm prolapse occurs when the cervix has dilated and the membranes rupture with the fetus in a transverse lie. The arm passes through the cervix and may be seen or felt protruding. An emergency caesarean section may be required.

arrested labour cessation in the progress of labour, possibly due to an obstruction.

artefact an artificially produced lesion.

arterial bleeding bleeding from an artery—identified by bright red blood and the pulsating nature of the flow.

arterial blood gas (ABG) the levels and pressures of oxygen and carbon dioxide in the blood of an artery. Measured in the blood of the umbilical artery in high-risk cases where fetal hypoxia is suspected.

arterial line a catheter inserted into an artery to obtain a continuous reading of the arterial blood pressure; sometimes used following severe obstetric emergency involving maternal collapse.

arterial pH the measurement of the blood against the acid–alkaline balance.

arteriole a small artery.

arteriosclerosis degenerative changes in the arteries resulting in thickening of the walls and making them less receptive to peristalsis.

artery a vessel carrying blood away from the heart.

artery forceps an instrument with locked scissor-like handles and flat serrated blades; used to clamp a bleeding vessel or hold tissue during surgical procedures.

arthritis inflammation of joints.

articulate unification of one or more joints; movement of one or more joints together.

articulation of the pelvis the relationship in degrees between the plane of the pelvis with the horizontal plane and the spine.

artificial feeding feeding of a baby, other than with breast milk. Commonly referred to as formula feeding.

artificial insemination introduction of sperm into the uterus by mechanical means rather than by sexual intercourse to achieve fertilisation and pregnancy.

artificial respiration the maintenance of breathing by

mouth to mouth (or mouth to mouth and nose) from another person or by a machine.

artificial rupture of membranes (ARM) the membranes are punctured and amniotic fluid released; often carried out to speed up labour and to see if meconium has been passed indicating fetal distress; *see* amniotomy.

ascites collection of free fluid in the peritoneal cavity; usually associated with heart failure. When seen in the fetus it is associated with severe anaemia and hydrops fetalis.

asepsis the complete absence of microscopic organisms or bacteria.

aseptic technique a procedure undertaken using sterile equipment and technique so that microorganisms will not be introduced into the body.

asexual without reference to gender; without sex organs.

asoma a fetus without a complete trunk and head.

aspermatogenesis testicles that do not produce sperm.

aspermia failure of spermatozoa to mature.

asphyxia oxygen deprivation. *Asphyxia neonatorum* is failure of initiation of respiration in the newborn infant; blood oxygen levels are low and the carbon dioxide level is very high.

aspiration the process of drawing up of fluid or gases from a cavity by suction. Meconium aspiration occurs when meconium has been passed before birth and entered the lungs in utero or during the first few breaths after birth.

aspiration pneumonia pneumonia caused by inhalation of infected materials from the upper respiratory tract or gastric content; burning of the lung lining by acid drawn up from the stomach and then inhaled.

aspirator an implement which, when negative pressure is applied, is used to draw fluid or gas from a cavity.

assessing collecting information regarding situation, history, progress or behaviour.

assessment a statement of evaluation or appraisal of behaviour or progress towards a goal.

assimilation the conversion of absorbed food into the substance of the body.

assimilation pelvis a pelvic deformity where the transverse processes of the last lumbar vertebra are fused with the sacrum. An alternative is where the last sacral vertebra is fused with the first coccygeal body.

assisted breech an approach to assisting the birth of the baby presenting by the breech vaginally. The baby is born spontaneously as far as the umbilicus, but the remainder of the birth of the body is assisted by various manoeuvres and application of forceps for the birth of the aftercoming head.

assisted reproductive technology (ART) the branch of medicine which helps women/couples to conceive a baby.

assisted vaginal/instrumental birth vaginal birth using forceps or vacuum extraction.

asthma a respiratory condition in which there is muscle spasm causing narrowing of the trachea and bronchi, thus creating difficulties in breathing with accompanying cough and wheezing sound on expiration.

asymmetric two halves or parts of the same, which should look and behave the same but do not.

asymmetry lack of balance between two similar structures. One side is not the same as the other.

asynclitism the position of the fetal head within the pelvis where one of the parietal bones is further down than the other. Usually, the fetal head needs to move to a synclitic position in order to negotiate the pelvis. This can be achieved in practice by encouraging maternal asymmetrical positions.

atelectasis incomplete inflation of the lungs. This may be primary failure at birth or secondary to obstruction and collapse. Seen especially in preterm babies.

athetosis involuntary movements of the hands and feet and other body parts.

atlas the first cervical vertebra, which moves under the occipital bone.

atonic relating to, caused by or exhibiting lack of muscle tone. *atonic uterus*: uterus lacking in tone which will lead to excessive bleeding in the postpartum period.

atony absence of muscle tone.

atresia blind end or closure of a normally open canal. In the neonate it can be associated with the oesophagus or anus as a congenital abnormality.

atrial septal defect a congenital condition in which the septum of the heart is abnormal—usually there is a hole allowing communication between the left and right atria (*see* Fig. 8).

atrium (PLURAL atria) the singular name for the upper chambers of the heart.

atrophic vaginitis degeneration of the vaginal mucous membrane, usually after the menopause, leading to a reduction in size.

atrophy withered degeneration of cells leading to a reduction in their size.

atropine (hyoscyamine) an alkaloid extract of the belladonna plant (*Atropa belladonna*) which can be administered prior to surgery for reducing secretions of the gastrointestinal and respiratory tracts and to induce muscle relaxation.

attachment theory a highly specific type of social bond; a complementary, asymmetrical relationship in which one

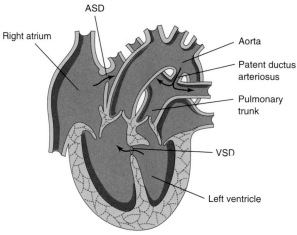

ASD

Right atrium

Aorta

Patent ductus
arteriosus

Pulmonary
trunk

VSD

Left ventricle

Figure 8
Atrial septal defect (ASD)

participant seeks comfort and
safety from the other.
attitude relating to position or
posture. The relationship of
the fetal parts to each other,
e.g. head to spine.
atypical differing from what
might normally be expected.
audio- combining form
meaning associated with the
sense of hearing. *Auditory* has
the same meaning.
audit a means of evaluating
care and its relationship to
research and expected
standards. Changes can be
made as a result to enable

expected standards to be
achieved.
augment to accelerate or
intensify an established
process, as in the use of
oxytocin in a labour that is
slow to progress.
augmentation a procedure in
which a substance is given to
stimulate or accelerate a
normal physiological process.
aura a warning sensation
experienced by a person with
epilepsy before a seizure.
aural relating to the ear.
auricle the external part of
the ear.

auscultation the process of listening to the sounds emitted by internal organs; listening to the fetal heartbeat in pregnancy.

authentic the quality of being open and honest in behaviour and motives; genuine or original.

autoclave a machine that sterilises equipment using steam under pressure. A gauge automatically regulates the pressure and the heat to which the contents are subjected.

autogenesis self-generation; origination within the organism.

autohypnosis the ability to induce a trance in oneself, and to become unaware of the world around. Some women use self-hypnosis to enable them to cope with the pain of labour.

autoimmune disease occurs when there is an overactive immune response to substances and tissues that are normally present in the body.

autoinfection self-infection.

autolysis (self-ingestion) the spontaneous breakdown of body tissues by enzymes. The uterine size is reduced to a non-pregnant size by this process during the 6 weeks after birth.

autonomic involuntary or independent of one's will or control, as, for example, the functioning of the *autonomic nervous system*.

autonomic nervous system the part of the nervous system which regulates smooth or involuntary muscles. The sympathetic nerves speed up contractions and gland secretion and increase muscle tone. The parasympathetic nerves reverse these processes.

autonomy right of self-government; in midwifery, this usually means the ability of the midwife to practise on her own responsibility for providing care for women in normal pregnancy and childbirth.

autopsy (SYNONYM postmortem) examination after death to determine the cause or improve understanding of disease progression.

autosomal dominant inheritance the gene-carrying markers for a specific disease will cause that condition even in the presence of a healthy paired partner.

autosomal recessive inheritance two affected genes need to have been inherited for the medical condition to be manifested, e.g. phenylketonuria.

autosome a chromosome that is non-sex determined.

autozygous genes which are copies of ancestral genes and the result of a consanguineous union.

avascular not vascular, bloodless.

average a value which is representative of a series of

numbers or items. The *mean average* is calculated by adding the sum of a series of numbers and dividing it by the number of items in the series; the *mode* (most frequently occurring number or item) and the *median* (central number when all are placed in order) *averages* may also be used.

axilla (SYNONYM armpit) the hollow depression beneath the arm and chest.

axillary pertaining to the axilla.

axillary node a lymph gland found in the armpit.

axillary tail of Spence breast tissue that extends to the armpit.

axillary temperature the body temperature recorded by placing a thermometer under the armpit.

axillary traction a maneuver by which the fingers of the birth attendant are used to free the baby's shoulder during a shoulder dystocia.

axis an imaginary line passing through the centre of the body; the second cervical vertebra, over which the atlas moves.

axis traction the process of pulling on the fetal head to aid delivery when progress in the second stage of labour is arrested.

azoospermia absence of spermatozoa in semen.

Bb

B one of the antigens found on red cells, present in human blood groups B and AB.

Babinski's reflex a normal reflex in the newborn in which the great toe extends and the other toes fan out when the lateral aspect of the foot is stroked.

Baby Friendly Health Initiative (BFHI) aims to give every baby the best start in life by creating a healthcare environment where breastfeeding is the norm. Launched by the World Health Organization (WHO) and United Nations Children's Fund (UNICEF) in 1991. It has also been called the Baby Friendly Hospital Initiative.

bacillary rod-shaped; relating to a bacillus.

bacille Calmette-Guérin (BCG) an attenuated (weakened) strain of tubercle bacillus used in vaccines to immunise against tuberculosis.

bacilluria the presence of bacilli in the urine.

bacillus (PLURAL bacilli) a generic term for any rod-like bacterial organism; a bacterium of the genus *Bacillus* (family Bacillaceae).

backache pain located over the lumbar region of the back; occurs frequently in pregnancy due to changes in the centre of gravity as the uterus becomes heavier.

bacteraemia presence of bacteria in the blood.

bacteria (SINGULAR bacterium) a group of single-celled microscopic organisms universally found in plants and animals. Some of these can be disease-forming when they enter the body. Others can be protective.

bacterial shock a state of shock with severe hypotension and circulatory failure resulting from bacteraemia.

bacterial vaginosis (BV) occurs when the amount of normal *Lactobacillus* species in the vagina is deficient, affecting the normal acidity of the vagina and allowing a relative overgrowth of anaerobic bacteria.

bactericide an agent that destroys bacteria.

bacteriology the scientific study of bacteria.

bacteriostatic an agent capable of arresting bacterial growth.

bacteriuria presence of bacteria in the urine. May be asymptomatic in pregnancy.

bag of waters (*slang*) common term some women may use for the liquor contained in the fetal membranes.

Bakri® balloon tamponade a surgical intervention that may be used to treat severe postpartum haemorrhage. It consists of a silicone balloon that is placed inside the uterus to control bleeding.

balanic refers to the glans penis in the male and the clitoris in the female.

balanitis inflammation of the glans penis. In babies it may indicate the need for more frequent changes of nappy.

ballottement a diagnostic procedure used to determine the presence of a floating organ or object such as a fetus. The object or organ is pushed or tapped to encourage displacement and rebound of content against the containing wall such that the impact is palpable.

Bandl's ring the pathological thickening of the normal retraction ring that occurs when labour is obstructed. If it is palpable abdominally, it is an indication of imminent uterine rupture.

barbiturates a group of drugs acting on the brain to produce a hypnotic and sedative effect.

bariatrics the study of overweight, its causes, prevention and treatment.

Barlow's test a test done to diagnose congenital dislocation of the hips.

baroreceptor in the walls of the body's major arteries are receptors which are stimulated by changes in blood pressure. The signals from these baroreceptors may lead to changes (usually a reduction) in arterial blood pressure.

barrier nursing the care of infectious people in isolation from other patients to avoid infecting others with an illness unrelated to their original one.

bartholinitis inflammation of a Bartholin's gland. Can result in cystic or abscess formation.

Bartholin's glands glands situated on either side of the lower part of the vagina which produce alkaline secretions that assist in lubricating the vagina.

basal metabolic rate (BMR) a measure of the units of energy and oxygen used for production of heat by the body at rest. It is expressed as a percentage above or below that used by others of the same height, weight and age. In pregnancy the BMR is increased by up to 30%.

basal temperature the body's temperature is taken after rest and before rising. A rise of 0.5°C above the normal body temperature at the same time indicates that ovulation is imminent; the temperature will remain increased until the next menstrual period. Used as a means of natural family planning, sometimes in combination with other methods.

base the main component of a mixture; the bottom (e.g. the inferior aspect of the skull).

baseline fetal heart rate the mean level of the fetal heart rate (FHR) when this is stable, excluding accelerations and decelerations; expressed in beats per minute (bpm).

basophil a leucocyte with an affinity for basic dyes making them easier to examine.

battledore placenta a placenta in which there is displacement of the umbilical cord from the centre to the side.

BCG *see* bacille Calmette-Guérin.

b.d. (LATIN *bis die*) twice daily. Used in prescribing to indicate how often to give medicine.

bearing down describes both the sensation and the action of the expulsive contractions experienced during the second stage of labour, where the woman pushes, involuntarily or with added effort, in order to move her baby through the birth canal.

bed rest curtailment of all ambulatory activities and restriction to rest in bed.

Bell's palsy paralysis of the face caused by facial nerve damage; this may be as a result of trauma during a forceps delivery, shoulder dystocia, exposure to cold or viral infection.

benign non-malignant; not dangerous to life.

best practice in maternity care aims to ensure that women and newborns receive quality care that is safe, effective and based on the best available evidence.

beta (β) denoting second. Often combined with the name of another substance or compound.

beta-haemolytic streptococcus a streptococcal bacterium that is potentially pathogenic and can be fatal to the neonate.

betamethasone a steroid offered to women when preterm birth is imminent or probable in order to promote fetal lung surfactant.

bi-, bin- prefix denoting two.

bicarbonate a salt of carbonic acid. Sodium bicarbonate is used to correct acidaemia.

bicornuate uterus congenital anomaly in which there is incomplete fusion of the two tubes which unite to form the uterus. The uterus is heart-shaped or has a septum (bicornuate or bicornate, having two horns; *see* Fig. 9). Contractions are less efficient and placental retention is common.

bigeminal pregnancy a twin pregnancy.

bilateral referring to both sides of the body.

bile a bitter greenish alkaline substance secreted by the liver whose function is to aid breakdown and absorption of fats in the intestines.

bilirubin a product resulting from the breakdown of haemoglobin. It is the main pigment found in bile. It is insoluble in water, but once conjugated by the liver it can

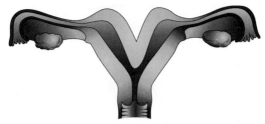

Figure 9
Bicornuate uterus

be excreted in faeces and urine. In neonatal life the liver is immature and haemolysis is excessive. The bilirubin will remain fat-soluble and be stored in the skin which will subsequently appear yellow (jaundiced).

bilirubinaemia high levels of red/orange bile pigment circulating in the blood. Very high levels will stain fat yellow in the brain and may cause permanent damage (kernicterus).

bilirubinometer an instrument for measuring the concentration of bilirubin in blood.

Billings method a means of determining the fertile period in the menstrual cycle by examination of the consistency of cervical mucus; the mucus becomes stretchy around the time of ovulation.

bimanual using both hands, as in *bimanual palpation*, an examination performed using two hands.

bimanual compression of the uterus a method used to arrest severe postpartum haemorrhage by squeezing the uterus. One hand is externally placed abdominally over the uterine fundus and the other formed into a fist anterior fornix of the vagina. The clinician compresses the uterus between the two hands (*see* Fig. 10).

bimanual palpation of the pelvic organs examination of the pelvic organs with one hand over the lower abdomen and two fingers of the other hand in the vagina (*see* Fig. 11). Used for early pregnancy detection.

binary gender the classification of gender into the two categories of either man or woman based on biological sex. *See also* non-binary.

binovular derived from two separate ova, as in binovular twin pregnancy.

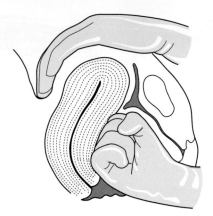

Figure 10
Bimanual compression of uterus

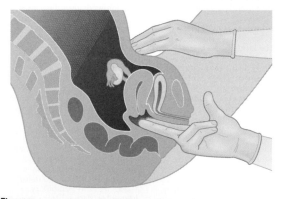

Figure 11
Bimanual palpation of the pelvic organs

biochemistry the study of the chemicals, elements and their reactions within living tissues.

biological profile *see* biophysical profile.

biophysical profile (BPP) is a non-invasive test that predicts the presence or absence of fetal asphyxia using ultrasound measurements, most commonly measurement of the amniotic fluid index (AFI), observation of the presence or absence of fetal breathing movements, gross body movements, and tone.

biopsy the excision of tissue from a living body and its use for diagnostic study.

biorhythm (biologic rhythm) the established regularity with which certain phenomena recur in living organisms, such as a circadian rhythm.

biparietal diameter the measured distance between the parietal eminences of the fetal skull, made by the use of ultrasound scan. Used to estimate fetal growth and maturity and traditionally taken as 9.5 cm at term.

biparous a woman who has given birth to two infants in different pregnancies.

bipartite having two parts; a placenta can be called bipartite if there are two parts, not necessarily of equal size.

bipolar having two poles. A term commonly applied to the pregnant uterus.

bipolar disorder a mental health condition previously known as manic-depressive illness. It is often characterised by unusual shifts in a person's mood and level of energy for activities of daily living.

birth the process by which the baby, and the placenta and membranes, are expelled via the birth canal.

birth asphyxia failure of the baby to initiate spontaneous respirations at birth.

birth canal a collective description of the birth passage which includes the soft and bony structures traversed by the baby during vaginal birth.

birth centre home-like setting in which women can labour and give birth. Some birth centres are *freestanding*, that is, they are geographically separate from a maternity unit. Others are *along-aside*, which means it is within the campus of the maternity unit or hospital. Many birth centres provide women with midwifery continuity of care through pregnancy, birth and the early postnatal period.

birth certificate a legal document recording details of a person's date and place of birth, gender, given name and names of parents; used as a form of identification.

birth control methods used in the regulation and avoidance of conception.

birth defect any structural defect or chromosomal

abnormality detected during pregnancy, at birth or in the first year of life.

birth injury damage such as intracranial haemorrhage, and brachial plexus nerve damage sustained by the fetus during birth.

birth mother the woman who gives birth to the baby, but not necessarily the genetic mother.

birth notification the requirement to give information of a birth to the appropriate authority within a stipulated timeframe.

birth plan a description by the woman of care she would like in labour.

birth rate also known as births per population rate. It is the total number of live births per 1000 of a population in a year.

birth registration the legal requirement that all births be registered.

birth trauma injury occurring during birth; may be mild or severe, and injuries may be temporary or permanent and encompasses physical as well as psychological trauma.

birth weight the newborn infant's first bare weight in grams. Low birth weight: birth weight less than 2500 g. Very low birth weight: birth weight less than 1500 g. Extremely low birth weight: birth weight less than 1000 g.

birthing chair chair designed to give the advantages of the upright position for the second stage of labour.

birthing on country a metaphor for the best start in life for Australian Aboriginal and Torres Strait Islander babies and their families, which provides an appropriate transition to motherhood and parenting, and an integrated, holistic and culturally appropriate model of care for all.

birthing stool crescent-shaped stool on which a woman may sit for support during labour and birth.

birthmark a skin blemish present at birth; it may be either a pigmented naevus or a vascular haemangioma.

bisacromial diameter a measurement of the distance between the acromion processes of the shoulder blades. In the term fetus the bisacromial diameter measures approximately 12 cm.

bisexual possessing both male and female characteristics; in adults, a person who is sexually attracted to both women and men.

Bishop's score a method of assessing the condition of the cervix and its favourability for induction of labour. An unfavourable cervix may be ripened by the administration of prostaglandin gel or pessaries prior to induction.

bitemporal diameter measurement of the diameter between the coronal sutures taken at the inferior end, usually 8.2 cm at term.

bitrochanteric diameter the measured distance between the greater trochanters of the femur taken just below the neck. It is the engaging diameter when the fetus presents by the breech and is usually 10 cm at term.

bladder the hollow muscular sac that is a reservoir for urine.

blastocyst the primitive and early differentiation of the conceptus. It consists of trophoblast, inner cell mass and blastocoele.

blastoderm the layer of cells formed by the cleavage of a fertilised mammalian egg. It later divides into the three germ layers from which the embryo develops.

blastula an early stage in the development of a zygote as it progresses to become an embryo.

blastulation the transformation of the morula into a blastocyst.

bleed to lose blood from the circulation.

bleeding time the time taken to stop bleeding; 1–9 minutes in the non-pregnant state.

blighted ovum an abnormal ovum which grows, but not into an embryo.

blister a collection of serum between the epidermis and the true skin.

block an obstruction. *Epidural block* occurs when the passage of impulses up the spinal cord has been stopped by local anaesthetic in the epidural space.

blood bank a refrigerated storage facility where blood for future transfusion is kept.

blood cell can be *red blood cells* (erythrocytes) or *white blood cells* (leucocytes).

Modified Bishop's scoring system (to assess favourability of cervix for induction of labour)				
Assessment features	0	1	2	3
Dilatation of the cervix (cm)	0	1–2	3–4	5–6
Consistency of the cervix	Firm	Medium	Soft	–
Length of cervical canal (cm)	> 2	1–2	0.5–1	< 0.5
Position of cervix	Posterior	Mid	Anterior	–
Station of presenting part related to ischial spines	–3	–2	–3	+1, +2

When the total score is greater than eight, the cervix is said to be favourable.

Source: Adapted from Royal College of Obstetricians and Gynaecologists. Induction of labour. Evidence-based Clinical Guideline No. 9. London: RCOG Press, 2001.

blood cross-matching a test to assess compatibility of blood before transfusion. Recipient serum is mixed with donor cells or donor serum with recipient cells. If agglutination does not occur the blood is deemed compatible.

blood gases the concentration of oxygen, carbon dioxide and bicarbonate in the blood. Measured in fetal or cord blood in neonates at risk of having suffered occult asphyxia.

blood group genetically determined classification of human erythrocytes based on the presence of specific antigens (agglutinogens) in the erythrocyte and antibodies (agglutinins) in the serum. Erythrocytes may also contain the Rh factor. People whose red blood cells contain antigen are classified as Rh-positive and those without the antigen as Rh-negative.

blood patch *see* epidural blood patch.

blood pH a measure of the acidity or alkalinity of blood. The average adult blood pH is 7.4.

blood pressure (BP) the pressure exerted by the blood on the vessel wall. When being measured as a screening or diagnostic procedure two measurements are taken. The first measurement, or systolic, is the maximum pressure within the brachial artery during contraction of the ventricles and the second, diastolic, the pressure within the artery when the ventricles are at rest.

blood sugar the amount of sugar (usually glucose) in the blood. The quantity varies and may rise following a meal and fall during fasting.

blood transfusion the taking of blood from one individual and administering it to another.

blood urea the quantity of urea in the blood—usually 2–6 mmol/dL.

blood volume the total quantity of blood in the body.

blue baby a baby who remains centrally cyanosed after establishment of respiration at birth. Cyanosis may be due to a severe cardiac or pulmonary abnormality.

body image the conscious or unconscious perception a person has of their body. This may change in pregnancy, depending on the woman's attitude to being pregnant, and may be reflected in her behaviour and her feelings about herself.

body mass index (BMI) (*see* Appendix 6) the relationship of weight to height expressed numerically. BMI scale: underweight = under 18.5; average = 18.5–24.99; overweight = 25–29.99; obese = 30 and over. Calculated BMI is determined by your weight in kg divided by your height in metres squared (kg/m^2).

body temperature heat produced by the body as a result of fuel metabolism. It is essential to maintain a stable environment for optimal functioning. In pregnancy the basal temperature may rise and the woman may feel warmer than people around her.

bonding the emotional attachment and dependence

between a mother and her baby/child. Initiated at birth, bonding can be interrupted where mother and baby are unnecessarily separated, or where medical or midwifery procedures are carried out which disturb mother–baby contact.

bone marrow a substance found in the hollow cavities of the bones.

booking the initial meeting between the healthcare provider and the pregnant woman, ideally before 12 weeks' gestation, when the woman's medical, family and obstetric history is recorded, needs for care are assessed, plans for care are drawn up, information is given and a relationship of trust is established.

borborygmus the rumbling sound produced by flatus in the intestine.

bowel the intestine.

bowel sounds sounds made by the movement of the intestines. Since the intestines are hollow, bowel sounds can echo throughout the abdomen. Bowel sounds are indicative that the intestines are functioning.

Bowman's capsule the glomerular capsule receiving the filtrate from the blood at the far end of the nephron in the kidney. It passes through the tubules where some reabsorption occurs.

brachial referring to the arm.

brachial artery an artery originating in the axilla

(armpit) that is palpable as it runs near the surface and anterior to the elbow, branching at the elbow to supply the radius and ulna.

brachial plexus nerves just above the clavicle which can become overstretched during a breech or vaginal delivery resulting in Erb's paralysis or Klumpke's paralysis.

brachycephaly a congenital abnormality in which the coronal sutures on the skull close early in development and the head expands sideways in order for the brain to develop.

brachydactylia abnormally short fingers.

bradycardia an abnormally slow heart rate—below 60 beats per minute in an adult, or below 90 beats per minute in a fetus.

brain the main part of the central nervous system contained within the cranium and consisting of the cerebellum, cerebrum, pons and medulla oblongata.

Brandt-Andrews manoeuvre manoeuvre for delivering the placenta and membranes after separation. One hand holds the uterus while the other puts traction on the cord. Should not be carried out during physiological third stage.

Braxton-Hicks contractions painless, intermittent contractions of the uterus occurring in pregnancy from 20 weeks' gestation.

breakthrough bleeding loss of blood from the uterus not associated with menstruation or pregnancy.

breast one of the two mammary glands situated on the anterior chest wall.

breast abscess infection and pus formation during lactation or weaning.

breast milk the nutritious substance secreted by the mammary glands; it appears 3–5 days after parturition following the secretion of colostrum.

breast milk jaundice jaundice which starts in the first few weeks of life as a result of a substance (metabolite) in the mother's milk that inhibits the infant from conjugating bilirubin to a glucuronide which can be excreted. The jaundice is mild and may correct itself or remain for the duration of breastfeeding. It is not a contraindication to breastfeeding.

breast pump apparatus for suctioning milk from the breast using hand or electric pumping action.

breastfeeding nourishing a baby by feeding milk from the breast(s).

breech the buttocks; the position when the fetus lies with its buttocks occupying the lower pole of the uterus (*see* Fig. 12).

breech extraction the assistance which may be provided at the birth of an infant being born vaginally. The accoucheur may exert

traction on the body or apply forceps to the aftercoming head. *See also* physiological breech birth.

breech presentation the baby lies in the uterus with its buttocks or feet presenting first.

bregma the anterior fontanelle. The larger of the two fibromembranous regions on the fetal skull found at the junction of the frontal, coronal and sagittal sutures.

brim of the pelvis the circumscribed inlet to the bony part of the birth canal.

broad ligaments a double fold of peritoneum extending laterally from the uterus to the pelvic wall and enclosing the fallopian tubes (*see* Fig. 13).

bronchopneumonia infection in the lungs with exudates settling in the bronchi and alveoli. May result from inhalation of meconium at birth.

bronchopulmonary dysplasia granular damage to the lungs associated with administration of high quantities of oxygen therapy in neonates with respiratory distress syndrome.

bronchus one of the primary branches of the trachea.

brow the upper anterior part of the head; forehead.

brow presentation when the fetus is a cephalic presentation, but the head is neither fully flexed nor fully extended (*see* Fig. 14). The

(a) Complete or full breech

(b) Frank breech

(c) Footling or incomplete breech

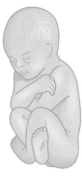

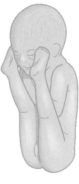

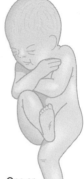

Fully flexed fetus

Not fully flexed fetus with legs extended

One or both thighs extended

Figure 12
Breech

mento-vertical diameter (which at 13.5 cm is larger than any of the pelvic diameters) presents, which can lead to an obstruction of labour and cephalopelvic disproportion.

brown fat a type of adipose tissue, a particularly easily accessible energy store. Only found in the newborn baby, between the shoulder blades, neck, around the sternum and kidneys. This fat is peculiar to the newborn and is usually metabolised within the first few weeks of birth.

Brushfield's spots small white spots on the edge of the iris of the eye. They may be associated with Down syndrome.

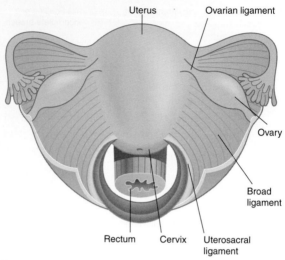

Figure 13
Broad ligament

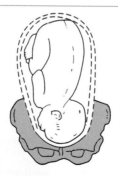

Figure 14
Brow presentation

buccal referring to the cheek; some drugs may be administered into the *buccal pouch* from where they are easily absorbed across the mucous membrane into the bloodstream.

buffer a chemical substance which, when present in a solution, helps to resist a change in pH.

bulbocavernosus muscles of the pelvic floor which encircle the vaginal orifice.

Burns-Marshall technique an older method of delivering the aftercoming head in a breech presentation. The baby's ankles were held and slight traction exerted as the feet were carried through a wide arc up to and over the mother's abdomen. Has been shown to be potentially hazardous and should no longer be used.

bundle a structured approach to the provision of effective care using a structured and clearly defined package of interventions. *See also* care bundle.

buttonholing a term applied to the appearance of the perineum as it is distended by the fetal head in the second stage of labour. The skin starts to tear along and within the perineal body indicating that a laceration will occur.

Cc

C symbolic representation for carbon.

C, c symbol used to denote Rh blood types, others being D, d and E, e.

caecum the part of the large intestine which contains the appendix.

caesarean section surgical incision into the abdominal and uterine wall to achieve birth of the baby (*see* Fig. 15).

caked breast a state of extreme engorgement of the breasts in which they become hard as the milk comes in and is not removed.

calcaneum (SYNONYM calcaneus) the heel bone.

calcaneus valgus a type of talipes in which the ankle is flexed and only the heel touches the ground.

calcification deposition of calcium salt within body tissues; calcification of the mature placenta. The degree of calcification of the fetal bones is used to denote maturity.

calcium a metal with a strong affinity for oxygen; widely found in nature.

calcium phosphate one of three calcium salts. Essential to the formation of strong bones and teeth.

calcium supplementation additional calcium intake, usually in the form of tablets, that may be taken by pregnant women.

calculus (stone) a solid collection of mineral substances; may be found in the kidneys or gall bladder and requires surgical removal if symptoms of obstruction occur.

Caldwell-Moloy pelvic classification a system used for classifying the female pelvis as one of four types: gynaecoid, android, anthropoid and platypelloid.

calipers curved, hinged compasses for measuring the diameter of convex bodies, e.g. the fetal skull.

callus new growth of bone tissue which forms at the margin of fractures as part of the healing process.

calorie a unit of heat or amount of fuel needed to raise the temperature of 1 g of water by 1°C.

cancer a general term to describe malignant growths.

Candida (*Candida albicans*, *Monilia albicans*) a fungus or yeast-like pathogen causing thrush.

candidiasis fungal infection found in the vagina, mouth and sometimes on the skin around the nipple. The neonate can be infected during breastfeeding.

canker sore an ulcer-like lesion on the genitals or in the mouth.

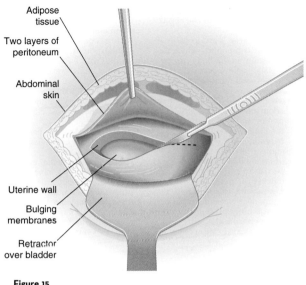

Figure 15
Caesarean section layers

Adipose tissue
Two layers of peritoneum
Abdominal skin
Uterine wall
Bulging membranes
Retractor over bladder

---

cannabis the flowering top of the hemp plant used to treat glaucoma and nausea and which can create an altered state of consciousness.

cannula an artificial tube inserted into the body cavity for delivery of drugs or fluids, or to enable drainage of fluids. It is often fitted with a trocar for insertion.

cannulation the insertion of a cannula (narrow patent tube) into the body.

cap contraceptive diaphragm which covers the cervix to prevent entry of sperm; often used with a spermicide.

capillary minute, hair-like vessels connecting arteries, veins or the lymphatic system.

capillary haemangioma a birthmark on the skin made of tiny blood vessels.

caput succedaneum oedematous swelling on the presenting part of the head, occurring during labour when venous return is restricted by tight application of the cervix (*see* Fig. 16).

carbohydrates a group of organic compounds which on ingestion by the body can be metabolised for energy, growth and repair of tissue.

carbonate a salt of carbonic acid.

carbon dioxide (CO₂) an odourless, colourless gas present in small quantities in the atmosphere. It is also a byproduct of tissue oxidation and is excreted via the lungs.

carbon dioxide tension the partial pressure of carbon dioxide gas in the blood. Its measurement usually reflects pulmonary gaseous exchange. The quantity present in blood obtained from the fetus or umbilical cord can indicate the degree of asphyxia or otherwise.

carbon monoxide a highly toxic gas produced by combustion. It has a high affinity with haemoglobin to which it binds, preventing uptake of oxygen. Present in the bodies of people who smoke cigarettes and those who passively inhale cigarette smoke.

carboprost a synthetic version of dinoprost, a prostaglandin; it has been used as a third-line management agent for postpartum haemorrhage, elective termination of pregnancy and miscarriage.

carboxyhaemoglobin the displacement of oxygen from erythrocyte and replacement with carbon dioxide.

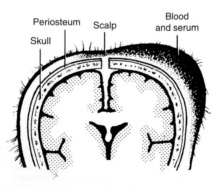

Figure 16
Caput succedaneum

carcinogen an agent which may cause a carcinoma to develop.

carcinoma a malignant tumour or uncontrolled growth of cells structurally and functionally different from and disruptive to those around them.

cardia the cardiac opening; the cardiac part of the stomach.

cardiac arrest cessation of heart contractions and failure of cardiac output. In labouring women this may be due to drug reaction, severe haemorrhage or other obstetric emergency.

cardiac massage rhythmic repeated downward pressure on the sternum to compress the heart and so maintain circulation.

cardiac output the amount of blood (expressed in litres) ejected by the left ventricle of the heart in 1 minute. Normal values are increased in pregnancy due to increased blood volume.

cardiac sphincter the round muscle between the stomach and the oesophagus. In pregnancy the muscle may be slightly relaxed allowing reflux of gastric juices into the oesophagus or mouth causing heartburn.

cardinal of first importance.

cardinal ligament (SYNONYM transverse cervical ligament) the lower thickened portions of the broad ligament which is firmly anchored to the cervix and lateral walls of the pelvis, providing support to the uterus.

cardinal movements of labour (SYNONYM mechanisms of labour) the principal positions and movements of the fetus during its passage through the birth canal.

cardiography an electronic recorded trace of heart movement and function.

cardiotocography (CTG) process of graphically recording the fetal heart rate pattern and uterine contractions.

cardiovascular pertaining to the heart and blood vessels.

cardiovascular shunt an abnormal communication between chambers of the heart and/or blood vessels. In fetal life a shunt between the atria is normal to bypass the pulmonary circulation. The shunt will normally close 6–48 hours after birth.

cardiovascular system the network of passages by which blood gases and nutrients are moved around the body.

care bundle a structured approach to the provision of effective care using a structured and clearly defined package of interventions. See also bundle.

caries decay, or necrosis of bone.

carneous mole the appearance of a fleshy mass surrounding a dead embryo.

carotid bodies a mass of specialised epithelioid tissue containing both baroreceptors and chemoreceptors found in blood vessels in the neck. They are sensitive to fluctuating oxygen content and trigger compensatory changes in respiratory rate, heart rate and blood pressure.

carpal relating to the wrist.

carpal tunnel syndrome symptoms of altered sensation such as pain and tingling due to compression of the median nerve at the wrist (*see* Fig. 17). This is usually due to trauma but in pregnancy may be due to pressure caused by the extra fluid in the circulation.

carrier 1. a person who is physically well but harbours an infective organism and is capable of transmitting it to others. 2. an individual who carries a mutant or recessive gene without manifestation of its defective characteristic.

cartilaginous joint immovable joint composed of cartilage; this includes the sacroiliac joint and the symphysis pubis. Under the influence of oestrogen and progesterone in pregnancy these joints will soften and separate, enlarging the pelvic diameters and causing instability and movement of the pelvic girdle.

caruncle a small fleshy mass.

carunculae myrtiformes tags of tissue that remain following rupture of the hymen membranes in the vagina.

casein a protein found in milk. The casein in cows' milk is more plentiful and less digestible than that in human milk.

caseload midwifery a way of organising midwifery practice where each midwife is responsible for the total care of a small group of women.

cast a structure moulded in a hollow organ and retaining the shape of the cavity of the organ when removed.

cat cry syndrome (SYNONYM cri du chat syndrome) a syndrome where the newborn has a particular cry suggestive of laryngeal problems; associated with chromosomal abnormalities.

cat eye syndrome vertical pupils (like those of a cat) seen in the newborn and associated with a chromosomal abnormality.

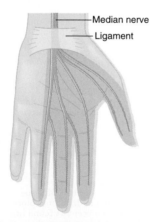

Median nerve
Ligament

Figure 17
Carpal tunnel syndrome

catabolism metabolism by the body of complex compounds for the production of energy.

cataracts clouding or opacity of the lenses or capsule of the eyes leading to impaired vision or blindness. Congenital cataracts may be familial or associated with maternal rubella during pregnancy.

catchment area geographical region served by a specific primary healthcare group or hospital, including the midwife.

catecholamines a group of hormones produced in response to stress; catecholamine production in labour can inhibit progress and lead to perceived 'failure to progress'.

catgut an absorbable material made from sheep's intestine used for closure of surgical wounds.

catheter a hollow tube made from various materials which may be introduced into a cavity to achieve drainage, e.g. a *urethral catheter* for bladder drainage.

catheterisation introduction of a catheter.

cathode a negative electrode.

Caucasian term often used to refer to people whose skin is white or very light and whose ancestors are thought to have inhabited the Caucasus region of south-eastern Europe.

cauda resembling a tail.

cauda equina the terminal branching filaments of the spinal cord which resemble a horse's tail.

caudal analgesia, caudal anaesthesia analgesia or anaesthesia achieved by injecting local anaesthetic solution into the sacral canal.

caul The baby is born in the membranous sac.

cautery sealing of torn blood vessels or coagulation of tissue by burning with a diathermy machine.

cavernous containing spaces or hollow areas.

cavity 1. hollow space. 2. lesion, as in dental caries.

cavity of the pelvis the region of the pelvis circumscribed by the brim, bony side walls and outlet.

CDH abbreviation for congenital dislocation of the hip.

-cele suffix denoting pathological swelling or tumour.

cell a singular structural and functional unit of a living organism that has the ability to grow and reproduce.

cell division a biological process of replication by mitosis, meiosis and amitosis.

cellulitis inflammation of tissue, usually the skin, due to infection or trauma.

cellulose a carbohydrate; the outer covering of vegetable cells.

Celsius scale scale of measurement for temperature—o°C is the freezing point of water and 100°C is the boiling point.

census an audit or survey conducted on an entire community to measure common factors so that future service needs can be anticipated.

Centering Pregnancy™ a model of antenatal care facilitated by a midwife and other health professionals that integrates health assessment, education and support within a stable group of women and families/friends.

centi- a prefix denoting a hundredth part.

central line a fine catheter inserted into a main vein (jugular) to diagnose a condition and administer fluids or medication; used following obstetric emergency such as postpartum haemorrhage, eclampsia or disseminated intravascular coagulation (DIC).

central nervous system (CNS) the brain and spinal cord.

central venous pressure (CVP) the filling pressure of the right ventricle used to regulate or monitor fluid replacement.

centre of gravity the midpoint or axis of rotation over which the weight of the body balances. In pregnancy the centre of gravity changes to accommodate the extra weight on the front of the abdomen; backache often results.

centrifuge an apparatus rotating at speed used for separating substances of different densities.

cephal-, cephalo- combining form meaning head.

cephalhaematoma a swelling on the neonatal head caused by a collection of blood beneath the periosteum.

cephalic presentation when the fetus adopts a head-down position in the uterus, the head will enter the pelvis first.

cephalic version turning of the baby to a head presentation by internal (ICV) or external (ECV) pressure from the operator's hands.

cephalocele a congenital abnormality in which the brain tissue protrudes through incompletely formed skull bone.

cephalometry the process of measuring the head.

cephalopelvic pertaining to the relationship between the fetal head and maternal pelvis.

cephalopelvic disproportion (CPD) a mismatch between the size of the maternal pelvis and the size of the fetal head—the head is too large and will not pass through the pelvis.

cephalopelvimetry an X-ray measurement of the fetal head in relation to the pelvis to ascertain whether the head is able to pass through. Rarely used in current practice.

cerclage encircling of a part with a ring or loop. Cervical cerclage is where a woman whose cervix is at risk of early opening may be encircled with suture material.

cerebellum the inferior part or hindbrain situated below the cerebrum and above the pons and medulla oblongata.

cerebral pertaining to or involving the cerebrum.

cerebral dysrhythmia a disturbance or irregularity in behaviour of a person's brain waves as measured using electroencephalography.

cerebral haemorrhage bleeding into the tissues of the brain.

cerebral palsy paralysis of various muscles and/or intellectual/sensory impairment as a result of damage to the brain; spasticity resulting from impaired neurological function.

cerebrospinal involving the brain and spinal cord.

cerebrospinal fluid (CSF) the fluid contained within the cerebral ventricles which bathes and cushions the brain tissues and spinal cord.

cerebrum the largest portion of the brain, occupying the upper part of the skull and consisting of left and right hemispheres.

cervical relating to the neck. In midwifery it denotes the neck of the uterus.

cervical canal the passage within the cervical muscles which permits escape of menstrual blood, entry of sperm and passage of the baby during birth. During pregnancy it contains a thick mucus plug called the operculum.

cervical cap a contraceptive device consisting of a small rubber cap which fits tightly over the cervix to prevent the penetration of sperm.

cervical dilation the opening of the cervical canal during labour to permit the baby to pass out of the uterus into the vaginal canal.

cervical erosion destruction of the squamous epithelial lining of the cervix by infection or trauma leaving abrasions which may bleed.

cervical intraepithelial neoplasia (CIN) the abnormal growth of precancerous cells in the cervix.

cervical polyp an overgrowth of cervical membrane forming a smooth regular mass within the cervical canal. It can also be on a stem which allows suspension into the vagina.

cervical smear scrapings of the secretions of cells from around the cervix for microscopic examination. Variations from the normal may indicate the beginning of a cancer.

cervicitis inflammation of the cervix, usually as a result of infection.

Cervidil (TRADE NAME) (dinoprostone, 10 mg) is a drug inserted vaginally to start and/or continue the ripening of the cervix in pregnant women for induction of labour.

cervix lower part of the uterus which protrudes into the vagina.

Chadwick's sign blue discolouration of the vulva and vagina as a result of venous engorgement associated with early pregnancy.

chancre the initial ulcerated lesion of syphilis formed at the site of inoculation.

Changing Childbirth Report a report published by the United Kingdom government in 1993 which contained an assessment of maternity services and recommendations for improving women's satisfaction and has been used throughout the world.

chemotherapy the treatment of illness by chemical means; that is, by medication.

chest the thoracic cavity.

chemoprevention (also chemoprophylaxis) the use of medication for the purpose of preventing disease or infection.

chi square test (Greek *chi*, χ) a statistical test used to show the relationship between observed and expected data represented by frequencies. The test shows the probability of the data having occurred by chance.

chignon the large artificially created caput succedaneum associated with vacuum delivery (*see* Fig. 18).

childbearing period the time in a woman's life between the menarche and the menopause when she is naturally capable of producing children.

child protection concerned with requirements to ensure the safety of children in the community. Most countries have particular legislation and guidelines as to the responsibilities of midwives and other healthcare providers in relation to official reporting where there are concerns about the safety of the child. This may also be unborn children.

chiropractic a therapy using manipulation to treat diseases caused by abnormal function of the nervous system and abnormality in the spinal column.

Chlamydia member of the genus *Chlamydia*; a microorganism which resembles but is not a gram-negative bacterium. It can cause conjunctivitis, lymphogranuloma venereum, and pelvic inflammatory disease and respiratory tract infections.

chloasma patchy hyperpigmentation often seen on the faces of pregnant women. Commonly distributed across the forehead, nose and cheeks.

chloride a salt of chlorine.

choanal atresia obstruction of the posterior nasal orifices.

chocolate cyst an ovarian lesion characteristic of endometriosis in which cysts are filled with degenerated blood.

cholecystitis inflammation of the gall bladder.

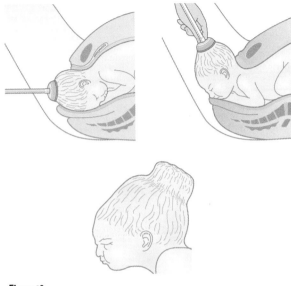

Figure 18
Chignon

chondroblast embryonic cell
that forms cartilage.
chordee downward curvature
of the penis caused by
congenital anomaly such as
hypospadias.
chorditis inflammation of
spermatic (or vocal) cords.
chorioadenoma destruens a
tumour of malignant
tendency, intermediate
between a hydatidiform mole
and a choriocarcinoma.

chorioamnionitis inflammation
of the chorionic and amnionic
membranes as a result of
bacterial invasion.
chorioangioma a common
tumour of the placenta
composed of fetal blood
vessels and connective tissue
in Wharton's jelly.
choriocarcinoma a
fast-growing tumour
originating from layers of
cytotrophoblast and

syncytiotrophoblast. Metastases occur through the blood and lymphatic system.

chorion the outermost fetal membrane which is in contact with the uterine cavity.

chorionic gonadotrophin a water-soluble hormone originating in chorionic tissue of the blastocyst and excreted in the urine of pregnant women. Its presence is diagnostic of pregnancy.

chorionic plate the part of the fetal placenta formed by merger of the trophoblastic layer and an internal lining of mesoderm from which villi grow into the lining of the uterus in very early pregnancy.

chorionic villi tiny vascular projections arising from the trophoblast which grow into the maternal blood sinuses. They absorb oxygen and nutrients to supply the demands of the growing conceptus.

chorionic villus sampling a procedure attended under ultrasound guidance to collect a small sample of chorionic villus (developing placenta) for examination of chromosomes or specific genes (*see* Fig. 19).

choroid plexus the vascular projections which extend into the ventricles of the brain from which cerebrospinal fluid is derived.

Christmas disease *see* haemophylia B.

chromatid one of two sister chromosomes, resulting from longitudinal division in preparation for mitosis.

chromosome microscopic structures contained in the cell nucleus which carry hereditary factors (genes). Each cell usually has 46 chromosomes except sperm and ovum which have 23 each.

chronic describes a condition which develops slowly and persists for a long time.

chronic hypertension (CH) The International Society for the Study of Hypertension in Pregnancy defines this as hypertension that is present in the preconception period, or the first half of pregnancy. It may be essential or secondary. Essential hypertension: blood pressure ≥ 140 mmHg systolic and/or ≥ 90 mmHg diastolic (K5) preconception or in the first half of pregnancy without an apparent underlying cause. It may also be diagnosed in those women presenting in pregnancy taking antihypertensive medications, again with no apparent underlying cause. Secondary hypertension: hypertension associated with renal, renovascular and endocrine disorders and aortic coarctation.

chronic hypertension and PE superimposed pre-eclampsia (PE) in women with underlying CH.

cilia hair-like cytoplasmic projections found on special epithelial cells; they beat

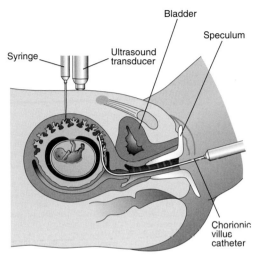

Figure 19
Chorionic villus sampling

rhythmically causing a current and enabling propulsion.

circulation movement in a defined circuit, e.g. *circulation of the blood*.

circulatory system the closed circuit or network of blood vessels, heart and lungs which supply the tissues of the body with all they need, remove waste, and carry microorganisms, cancer cells and drugs.

circumcision surgical removal of the foreskin of males. In females, also known as female genital mutilation (FGM) and defined as all procedures involving partial or total removal of the external female genitalia.

circumvallate surrounded by an elevation, as in *circumvallate placenta*, a placenta in which an overgrowth of chorionic membranes results in formation of a white ridge about the circumference.

cis/cisgender terms used to describe people whose gender corresponds to the sex they were assigned at birth.

clamp an instrument used to compress vessels or hollow organs to prevent bleeding, e.g. a *cord clamp* is used to clamp the umbilical cord after birth.

classical caesarean section delivery of the baby through a vertical incision made into the abdomen and the upper segment of the uterus.

clavicle the collarbone, a long bone between the sternum and the scapula. It may break or be broken (cleidotomy) if shoulder dystocia occurs in the second stage of labour.

cleft division or fissure.

cleft lip congenital defect resulting from failure of embryonic fusion of the median nasal and maxillary processes.

cleft palate congenital defect which usually accompanies cleft lip. The fissure may be partial or complete, allowing communication between the oral and nasal passages. The hard palate and gums may be absent or twisted.

cleidotomy breaking of the clavicle at the sternoclavicular joint to facilitate birth of the baby where there is obstruction due to the shoulders being too large.

climacteric the change of life; the menopause.

clinical assessment the evaluation of a person's physical condition; the theoretical application of knowledge to practice.

clitoridectomy the removal of part or all of the clitoris and a form of female genital mutilation (FGM). In some countries it is ritually performed on pubescent girls. It is considered to be an act of genital mutilation and is forbidden by law in many countries.

clitoris female erectile tissue, situated externally at the anterior junction of the labia minora and internally around the walls of the vagina. Once thought to be a homologue of the male penis, now known to be much larger and more intricate than previously realised.

clone a group of cells which are genetically identical, individually created by asexual reproduction and having identical genetic make-up.

clonic a term applied to the rapid involuntary muscular contraction and relaxation seen in seizures or fits.

Clostridium a bacterium of the genus *Clostridium*, a group of spore-forming anaerobic bacteria which cause gangrene, botulism, cellulitis and tetanus.

clot solidification of blood.

clotting time the time required for shed blood to clot under normal conditions.

club foot (talipes) *see* talipes.

CNS abbreviation for central nervous system.

coagulate to change from a liquid to a jelly-like mass.

coagulation clumping together of red blood cells.

coagulation factor one of the 12 substances in the blood which are required for the formation of a blood clot.

coarctation of the aorta stricture of the aorta at, or just below, the position of the ductus arteriosus.

coccus (PLURAL cocci) grain or seed—used to describe a microorganism of similar characteristic shape.

coccydynia persistent pain in the area of the coccyx.

coccygeal relating to the coccyx.

coccygeus one of the muscles of the pelvic floor arising from the ischial spines and anchored into the lateral borders of the sacrum and coccyx.

coccyx the lowest bone of the spinal column, formed by the fusion of four rudimentary vertebrae.

Cochrane Collaboration consists of systematic reviews on the effects of healthcare intervention published in the Cochrane Library.

coeliocolpotomy surgical entry into the abdomen gained through the vaginal wall.

cohort a group of people who share a common characteristic or experience within a defined time period; in common use for research enquiry.

cohort study a form of longitudinal study used in health and social science. It is one type of study design.

coitus sexual intercourse.

cold injury cellular damage and impaired function occurring as a result of exposure to cold environmental temperatures.

colic acute spasmodic abdominal pain. In infancy it can be due to overfeeding or swallowing of air resulting in bouts of crying.

coliform resembling *E. coli.*

collodion baby a baby born with skin resembling a scaly paper-like membrane.

colonised presence of microorganisms at levels that do not result in symptoms nor immune response. An example is seen in women with group B streptococcus in late pregnancy.

colostrum the first milk secreted by the breasts. It contains large quantities of cells, lactalbumin and lactoprotein.

colovaginal pertaining to the colon and vagina, as in *colovaginal fistula,* a fistula or abnormal opening between the two structures.

colpalgia pain in the vagina.

colpo- pertaining to the vagina.

colpocystitis inflammation of the vagina and urinary bladder.

colpocystocele protrusion of the urinary bladder into the vagina, usually through a weakness or fistula in the anterior vaginal wall.

colporrhaphy surgical suturing and repair of the vaginal wall.

colposcope an instrument with a lens and a light used to examine the vagina and cervix; a vaginal speculum.

colpotomy a surgical incision into the wall of the vagina.

columnar epithelium a type of epithelium containing cylindrical cells.

commensal an organism which lives on another without harming it.

communicating hydrocephalus hydrocephalus in which there is ventricular communication due to either excess or extra cerebrospinal fluid being produced or poorly reabsorbed.

compatibility the ability to coexist harmoniously.

compensation the process of increasing efficiency in one physiologic structure to restore balance to a system, structure or body when another aspect of that system has failed.

competence the skills, knowledge and attitudes required for safe practice.

competences (competencies) statements accepted by professional midwifery organisations and often used to regulate midwifery practice.

competency element a component of competencies.

competency standards a way of describing competencies in statements that are measurable.

competency unit a component of competencies.

competent a person who is judged as having the skills, knowledge and attitudes required for safe practice.

complementary feeds feeds given to a neonate in addition to planned feeding regimen, whether breast or bottle feeds.

complementary therapy therapies and treatments that do not follow a dominant healthcare model but which can be used in conjunction with this approach. Examples include reflexology, herbal medicines, psychoprophylaxis, osteopathy, cranial osteopathy, relaxation therapy and acupuncture.

complete breech the baby is lying in utero with the knees and hips flexed or folded up and the buttocks presenting over the cervical os.

complete miscarriage the total expulsion of all products of conception.

complicated labour a labour in which there is a departure from the normal progress. Often referred to as complex in place of complicated.

complication a deviation from the normal or expected process.

compound presentation a complication of labour in which more than one part of the baby presents and may create an obstruction, e.g. head or arm.

concealed haemorrhage bleeding that is not obvious or cannot be seen, but which will cause deterioration in the condition of the individual and the vital signs.

conception 1. the mental, abstract formulation of ideas. 2. the fertilisation of the ovum by a spermatozoon.

conceptional age the age of the fetus in weeks from conception rather than from the last menstrual period—usually 2 weeks less.

conceptus refers to the fertilised ovum from the uniting of the gametes until birth.

condom a protective rubber sheath worn over the penis during sexual intercourse for preventing conception and cross-infection, especially with HIV.

condyloma a wart-like growth near the external genitalia or anus, which may occasionally be syphilitic in origin.

cone biopsy removal of a cone-shaped section from the cervix, performed to confirm diagnosis when a cervical smear test result suggests the presence of precancerous cells.

confinement 1. detention. 2. the period of childbearing or labour and the puerperium. This is not a preferred term for childbearing women.

confluence of the sinuses the wide junction or point of merger of the superior sagittal, straight and occipital sinuses with the large transverse sinuses; may cause bleeding into the brain and cerebral palsy may result.

congenital present at birth.

congenital dislocation of the hip (CDH) condition existing at birth where the hip joint is lax or the socket in which the head of the femur sits is shallow and the hips dislocate easily. Diagnosed by Barlow's test for hip instability and treated with splints.

congenital heart defect (CHD) structural defect of heart or great vessels, or both.

congenital infection infection acquired in utero, including rubella and cytomegalovirus.

congenital syphilis infection of a baby in utero due to placental transfer of the causative organism from a woman who has had syphilis during pregnancy. The neonate will have specific characteristics and intellectual and/or developmental impairment.

congestion abnormal accumulation of blood in a part of the body.

congestive dysmenorrhoea painful periods caused by extra blood in the vessels of the pelvis.

conjoined twins multiple pregnancy in which there has been incomplete cleavage of a single fertilised ovum. The twins remain partially joined together.

conjugata to bind or act together; referring to the conjugate diameters of the pelvis.

conjunctiva the mucous membrane lining the inner surface of the eyelids and covering the anterior aspect of the eye.

conjunctivitis inflammation of the mucous membrane lining the anterior aspect of the eyes and eyelids. In the neonate it may be due to infection acquired during passage through the vagina.

connective tissue tissue which binds together or

supports the structures of the body.

consanguinity a blood relationship between two people who then conceive a child.

consent permission given by people for tests and treatment to be carried out on them.

constipation delay in the passage of faeces which can cause pain and discomfort. Constipation is a common discomfort in pregnancy due to hormonal changes.

constriction ring a spasmodic contraction of uterine muscles leading to narrowing, usually at the junction of the upper and lower segments.

consumers users of maternity services, that is, the pregnant woman and her family.

contagion communication of disease from one person to another by direct contact.

contamination exposure of a sterile or clean fluid, tissue or person to pathogenic organisms.

continuity of midwifery care consistent philosophy or organisational structure underpinning the care provided by midwives across the antenatal, intrapartum and postpartum periods. Continuity of care can be provided in a variety of ways.

continuity of midwifery carer care by a midwife whom the woman has previously met, feels she has developed a 'relationship' with and believes she 'knows'.

continuous positive airway pressure (CPAP) a form of non-invasive artificial ventilation where the flow of air is delivered at a constant pressure. This prevents complete collapse of the alveoli after each breath. This is a common form of ventilation for babies who have respiratory distress syndrome.

contraception the prevention of conception.

contraceptive diaphragm a large rubber dome with a compressible outer ring which can be inserted into the vagina, often with spermicidal cream to prevent conception (*see* Fig. 20).

contraceptive method a measure designed to prevent sperm meeting ovum. Many methods are available and different methods suit different people.

contracted pelvis a pelvis in which any of the diameters are sufficiently shortened to interfere with the progress of labour.

contraction temporary shortening of muscle fibres. In labour this is accompanied by a degree of permanent muscle shortening during subsequent relaxation, retraction.

controlled cord traction method of delivering the placenta and membranes by putting tension on the umbilical cord after an oxytocic drug has been given by injection and the cord has

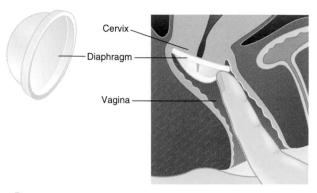

Figure 20
Contraceptive diaphragm

been clamped and cut (*see* Fig. 21).

controlled drug a pharmaceutical preparation whose prescription, administration, storage, dose, frequency of use and disposal is prescribed by statute because the drug may be misused or cause addiction.

convulsion an involuntary, generalised spasm of voluntary muscle fibres.

Cooley's anaemia thalassaemia.

Coombs' test test performed on cord blood to detect the presence of antibodies on the red cell surface. It is an indication of fetal/maternal incompatibility.

cord blood blood taken from the umbilical vein and/or artery just after birth.

cord presentation the umbilical cord is presenting at the cervical os; when the membranes are intact, continuation of labour may cause the fetal circulation to be impeded, with potentially fatal results for the baby (*see* Fig. 22).

cord prolapse the umbilical cord prolapses through the cervical os into the vagina (and possibly out of the introitus) in the presence of ruptured membranes. A potentially fatal condition for the baby which is usually treated by holding the presenting part up, thereby taking pressure off the cord, and offering immediate caesarean section.

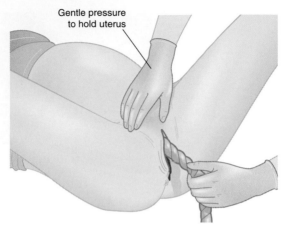

Gentle pressure
to hold uterus

Figure 21
Controlled cord traction

cordocentesis also sometimes called percutaneous umbilical blood sampling (PUBS), a technique used for both prenatal diagnosis and prenatal treatment of the fetus. Ultrasound is used to guide a thin needle directly through the woman's abdominal and uterine wall into the umbilical cord.

core midwives midwives based on the maternity unit usually working a roster system. Core midwives are usually based in one clinical area (antenatal, labour and birth, or postnatal).

cornea transparent part of the coating of the eyeball that covers the iris and pupil and admits light.

cornu (SYNONYM horn) the junction of the fallopian tubes with the uterus.

cornual pregnancy a pregnancy which has implanted in the narrow section of the fallopian tube as it enters the uterus. The pregnancy is not viable as the tube will rupture with severe bleeding by week 12—this is an emergency life-threatening situation requiring urgent surgery.

coronal suture the soft, fibrous, membranous region on the fetal skull between the frontal and parietal bones on each side of the skull.

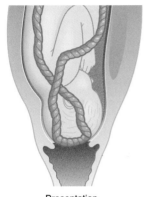
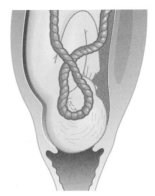

Presentation
of the cord

Occult presentation
of the cord

Figure 22
Cord presentation

coronavirus a group of related viruses that cause diseases in mammals and birds. Examples include rhinoviruses (common cold), as well as the viruses that cause SARS, MERS amd COVID-19.

corpus (SYNONYM body) the *corpus albicans* is the place on the ovary which has healed since the ovum escaped and the *corpus luteum* (formed after ovulation to produce oestrogen and progesterone) degenerated and stopped producing hormones.

corpus cavernosum spongy tissue in the penis or clitoris which becomes distended with blood during sexual arousal.

corpus luteum the yellow, blister-like follicle found on the surface of the ovary after expulsion of the ovum. It lives a short time and produces endocrine hormones; however, if pregnancy occurs its life is extended by the influence of human chorionic gonadotrophin.

corpuscle small body or cell.

cortex outermost layer of an organ.

cortical necrosis tissue death that results from blockage of the small arteries that supply blood to the outer part of the kidney (cortex) and causes acute kidney failure.

corticosteroid any of the hormones produced by the adrenal cortex.

cortisone one of several hormones produced by the adrenal cortex.

costal pertaining to the ribs.

cot death the unexplained death of an infant; *see* sudden infant death syndrome.

cotyledon a lobe or distantly separated group of placental villi supplied with blood vessels and supported by membranes.

couvade the mock labour sometimes experienced by men when their partner is in labour.

Couvelaire uterus bruised and purplish-blue discolouration of the uterus caused by blood escaping between the myometrial fibres. It is unable to contract because of the volume of blood within the tissues and so the placental site will continue to bleed unchecked.

COVAX a global initiative to ensure rapid and equitable access to COVID-19 vaccines for all countries, regardless of income level.

COVID-19 the disease caused by a novel coronavirus known as SARS-CoV-2.

cracked nipples associated with breastfeeding. The baby is not positioned correctly and the gums chew the lower margins of the nipple causing pain, cracking and bleeding.

cradle cap thick, yellow, greasy scales on the scalp of the infant.

cranial bones the bones of the skull (*see* Fig. 23).

cranial suture the fibromembranous structure found between the bones of the cranium in infancy.

craniodidymus a form of conjoined twins with two heads but fused bodies.

craniotabes defects and depressions found in the bones of the skull as the depositing of calcium in fetal life has not kept pace with cerebral development.

cranium skull.

creatinine a molecule that is generated from muscle metabolism as chemical waste. Creatinine is produced from creatine, which is important for muscles to produce energy.

credentialling a formal process used to verify and evaluate the qualifications and experience of healthcare professionals. It is a process often used by healthcare systems to assess the training, skills, experience and competence of individuals.

Credé's expression a rarely used method of assisting placental expulsion in which the uterine fundus is massaged to stimulate contraction, then squeezed.

cretinism a congenital condition in which the thyroid is deficient and a set of recognisable features are present including dwarfism and intellectual and/or developmental impairment.

cri du chat kitten-type mewing cry heard in the infant with neurological damage.

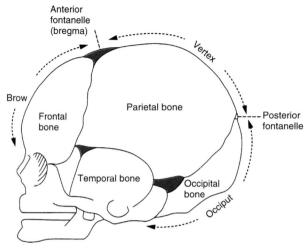

Figure 23
Cranial bones

---

cricoid pressure pressure applied to the cartilage of the larynx during induction of anaesthesia to protect the airway from gastric reflux.

criterion a standard which must be met and against which other standards or practices can be judged.

cross-infection the passing of pathogenic organisms from an infected person to a healthy one.

cross-matching of blood the procedure by which a donor's blood is mixed with that of a potential recipient to ensure

compatibility before a blood transfusion.

crowning when the suboccipitobregmatic and biparietal diameters of the fetal head distend the vulva and the head no longer recedes between contractions during the second stage of labour (*see* Fig. 24).

crown–rump length (CRL) ultrasonic measurement taken of the fetus during the first trimester to assess gestational age.

cryptodidymus conjoined twins, one being considerably

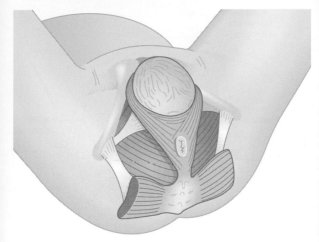

Figure 24
Crowning showing the pelvic floor muscles

---

smaller and developing within the body of the other.

cryptomenorrhoea subjective symptoms of menstruation without flow of blood.

culdocentesis removal of intraperitoneal fluids by aspiration with a hollow needle introduced through the vagina.

culdotomy surgical procedure performed via an incision into the pouch of Douglas through the vagina.

cultural safety an environment that ensures shared respect, meaning and knowledge and provides a space that is spiritually, socially and emotionally safe, as well as physically safe for people.

culture the propagation of microorganisms in a growth media.

curettage a surgical procedure in which a cavity is scraped clean (*see also* dilation and curettage).

curette a surgical instrument like a small spoon used for scraping the inside of hollow organs; used to clean the uterus of products of conception.

curriculum vitae (CV) a summary of a person's education, qualifications, professional experience, honours and activities sent to a prospective employer.

curve of Carus name given to the direction or pathway in which the fetal head moves to pass through the pelvis (*see* Fig. 25).

Cushing's syndrome the collection of symptoms and signs that are associated with an excess of the hormone cortisol.

cutaneous relating to the skin.

cyanosis blue discolouration of the skin and mucous membranes due to deficient oxygenation.

cyesis pregnancy.

cyst an enclosed pouch within tissue or organ, having a membranous lining, which is filled with fluid or other material.

cystic fibrosis a congenital disease in which mucous gland secretion is thick and obstructive. Malabsorption in the intestines and infection in the lungs are among the predominant features.

cystitis inflammation of the urinary bladder.

cysto- combining form denoting gall bladder, urinary bladder, pouch or cyst.

cystocele herniation of the urinary bladder into the vagina as a result of pelvic floor damage.

cystoscope an instrument for inspecting the interior of the bladder.

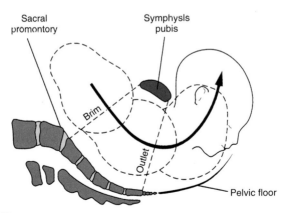

Figure 25
Curve of Carus

cystoscopy inspection of the interior of the bladder with a cystoscope.

cystotomy surgical incision of the urinary bladder.

cyto- pertaining to cells.

cytogenetics a branch of science in which cells and chromosomes are studied.

cytomegalovirus (CMV) a virus closely related to herpes. Infection of the fetus in utero may cause cytomegalic inclusion disease and result in an infant that may be small for gestational age, be jaundiced and suffer from liver disease.

cytoplasm the protoplasm of a cell other than the nucleus.

cytotoxic drug strong drug or chemical agent used to kill cancerous cells in the body. Such drug exposure during pregnancy will cause congenital abnormalities.

cytotrophoblast the inner cellular layer of the trophoblast.

Dd

D, d symbol denoting Rh blood group, others being C, c and E, e.

D&C *see* dilation and curettage.

dactyl digit.

day assessment unit (DAU) a place where screening and diagnosis can be done without the woman needing to stay overnight.

deceleration slowing down. In *fetal heart deceleration* the fetal heart rate falls below the accepted baseline rate.

decidua the lining of the uterus during pregnancy.

decidua basalis the part of the decidua beneath the implanted ovum.

decidua capsularis the part of the decidua which covers the implanted ovum.

decidual endometritis inflammation or infection of the decidua during pregnancy.

deciduoma a benign or malignant tumour in the endometrial tissue.

decreased fetal movements when women report less fetal movements than usual for their baby or report changes in the patterns of movements. Women with a concern about decreased fetal movements should be advised to contact their healthcare provider immediately.

deep transverse arrest the fetal head is unable to pass through the pelvis. It enters but cannot rotate or descend further.

deep vein thrombosis (DVT) a blood clot that forms in the muscle of the leg, usually the calf. Pregnant women are at risk due to changes in the clotting mechanism and immobility in labour or at caesarean section.

defecation the act of emptying the bowel.

deflexion a turning to one side; attitude of the fetal head when partially flexed.

deformity the condition of being distorted, flawed, malformed or misshapen.

degeneration destruction of cells resulting in impaired function.

degree 1. a unit of mathematical measurement, e.g. of temperature. 2. one of the intervals on a measuring tool, e.g. a thermometer. 3. an academic award conferred by a university or college.

dehiscence splitting open, as in the breaking down of a wound.

dehydration excessive loss of water from the body.

delay in labour prolongation of any of the three stages of labour.

delayed cord clamping (SYNONYM optimal cord clamping) umbilical cord clamping not earlier than 1 minute after birth as this has been shown to improve maternal and infant health and nutrition outcomes

delivery (SYNONYM birth) the expulsion of the baby, placenta and membranes. Not the preferred term; replace with birth e.g. *Estimated date of delivery should be estimated date of birth.*

delusion a false belief held by a person despite evidence against it.

demand feeding feeding the baby as and when it seems to be hungry, rather than at set times.

demography the study of populations and the incidence of disease, infection, etc.

denominator a defined point of the presenting part of the fetus which in relation to a given point on the mother's pelvis is used to indicate its position, occiput, mentum or sacrum.

deoxyribonucleic acid (DNA) a complex nucleoprotein found in chromosomes bearing coded genetic information and capable of reproduction in the presence of the appropriate enzyme.

dependence a state of being unable to function without that on which dependence is founded, e.g. a drug; a state of being reliant upon a person or substance.

depressant a drug which depresses or reduces the functioning of a system or of the whole body.

depression 1. a hollow or fossa. 2. a lowering of mood or state resulting in extreme sadness or dejection in which the person may be unable to carry out daily functions.

deprivation a state of being without the necessities for optimal physical, mental, social or spiritual wellbeing.

dermal referring to the skin or cutaneous layer.

dermoid cyst a benign cystic swelling containing skin and hair.

descent a movement downward. The term is applied to the presenting part of the baby as it moves through the pelvis towards the outlet. Assessed frequently in labour as it is an indicator of progress.

detachment separation or loss of anchorage of a structure from its support.

detrusor urinae muscle important fibres that form the outer layer of the urinary bladder. Because of the proximity to the vagina, damage can occur during childbirth which can result in incontinence.

development process of change and adaptation to a more advanced level of functioning.

developmental age an expression of a child's age when compared to a standard measurement.

developmental anomaly any abnormality or defect occurring before birth.

deviant a person who does not follow socially accepted standards of behaviour.

deviant behaviour actions contrary to those done by the majority of the community or culture.

deviation variation or turning away from a regular course or expected position.

dextral referring to the right side.

dextran a high-molecular-weight, water-soluble polysaccharide purified preparation which is used as a plasma expander for maintaining blood pressure and emergency treatment of shock.

dextro-, dextr- a combining term meaning favouring or turning to the right.

dextrocardia term meaning the heart is in the right half of the chest rather than the left.

dextrose a monosaccharide or sugar, the simplest form of carbohydrate.

di- prefix meaning two, twice.

diabetes insipidus a disease characterised by deficiency of antidiuretic hormone (vasopressin) resulting in excessive thirst and excretion of excessive volumes of dilute urine.

diabetes mellitus a condition where there is inadequate metabolism of carbohydrates and a disruption to the secretion of insulin process. Characteristic presentation is hyperglycaemia, glycosuria, polyuria, polydipsia, weight loss and ketoacidosis.

diabetic acidosis metabolic acidosis of uncontrolled diabetes in which there is an excess production of ketone bodies resulting from metabolism of body fats.

diagnosis identification of disease or state based on assessment of clinical symptoms.

diagnostic process systems used to indicate the nature of disease; follows on from a screening test.

diagonal any plane or straight line that is not vertical, perpendicular or horizontal; slantwise.

diagonal conjugate measurement of the internal pelvis, taken from the sacral promontory to the lower border of the symphysis pubis. In the normal pelvis it should measure 12.5 cm.

dialysis process using diffusion through a semipermeable membrane that can remove wastes or toxins from the blood and adjust fluid and electrolyte imbalances.

diameter a straight line passing through the centre of an object that joins points which go from one side to the other side of an organ, the pelvis or the fetal head.

diameters of fetal skull distances between certain landmarks on the fetal skull (*see* Fig. 26).

diaphragm shallow, dome-shaped cup with a flexible rim inserted into the vagina to prevent pregnancy.

diaphragmatic hernia embryonic development of the diaphragm in which there is persistence of the

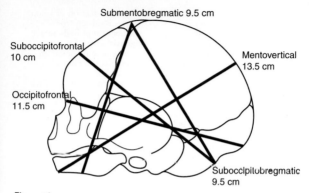

Figure 26
Diameters of fetal skull

pleuroperitoneal canal allowing part of the bowel to pass into the chest cavity (*see* Fig. 27).

diarrhoea frequent passage of loose, watery stools; often caused by a gastrointestinal infection.

diastasis separation of parts normally joined together, e.g. *symphysis pubis diastasis*.

diastole the resting phase of the cardiac cycle during which the chambers of the heart are dilated and fill with blood.

diastolic blood pressure the minimal measured pressure of blood felt in peripheral vessels during ventricular resting phase.

diathermy the applied therapeutic use of heat produced by high-frequency current to body tissue. Used to seal tissue together including bleeding vessels.

DIC *see* disseminated intravascular coagulation.

dicephalus a fetus with two heads.

didactylism only two digits on each hand.

didymus a testis.

dietician a health professional concerned with advising people about their eating patterns and offering nutritional advice.

differential diagnosis examination and comparison of signs and symptoms to

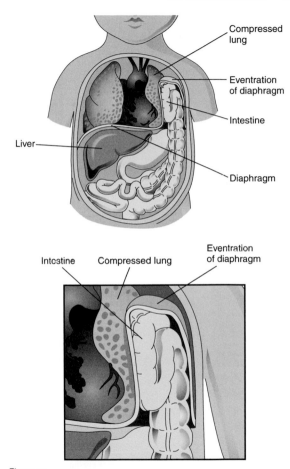

Figure 27
Diaphragmatic hernia

distinguish between diseases of similar characteristics.

differentiation unspecified cells are modified and organised to have specific characteristics and perform specific functions.

diffusion substances pass through a semipermeable membrane from an area of high concentration to one of low concentration.

digestion the process of breaking down into smaller parts or simpler compounds; the action of enzymes on ingested foods.

digestive juices enzymes found in the mouth and stomach which break down food. In pregnancy the stomach enzymes are more acidic than at other times and, if regurgitated, can cause burning of the mucous linings of the oesophagus; *see* Mendelson's syndrome.

digit a finger or toe.

dilatation (SYNONYM dilation) the process of stretching and opening, usually of a sphincter but also the cervix during labour.

dilation and curettage (D&C) widening of the cervix and scraping out (curettage) of the contents of the uterus; used to evacuate products of conception following incomplete abortion or as a diagnostic and therapeutic procedure in obstetrics and gynaecology (*see* Fig. 28).

dimorphism having the appearance of both sexes.

diovulatory two ova are released during one menstrual cycle.

diphtheria a rare but acute and potentially fatal infection against which a vaccine is offered during the first months of life.

diphtheria toxoid, tetanus toxoid and pertussis vaccine (DTP) combined immunisation.

diplococci (SINGULAR diplococcus) descriptive appearance of micrococci that always form pairs.

diploid having double quantities. Chromosomes have diploid numbers or 23 pairs.

diplopagus conjoined twins which are equally developed.

direct Coombs' test *see* Coombs' test; to detect antibody on red cell surfaces in umbilical cord blood.

direct endometriosis invasion of the myometrium by the mucous membranes lining the uterus.

disability a restriction in a person's ability to behave in a manner or within the range considered by the majority of the population as normal.

disaccharide a carbohydrate formed by condensation of two simple sugars.

discharge to emit, dismiss or release.

discharge summary report of events during hospitalisation sent to a person's general practitioner.

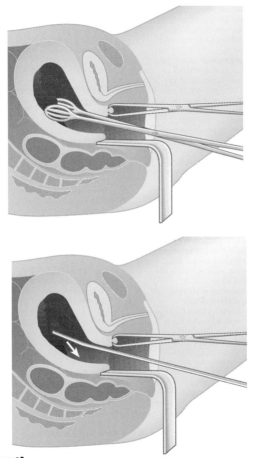

Figure 28
Dilation and curettage (D&C)

disease an abnormal condition caused by injury, infection or cancer resulting in a disturbance of normal bodily function.

disengagement emergence from a contained space; the manual removal of the fetal head or presenting part from the pelvis during caesarean section.

disinfect to destroy microorganisms by applying strong fluids or chemicals.

disjunction 1. moving apart or separation. 2. separation of homologous chromosomes at meiosis or mitotic division.

dislocation displacement of bone from its original position.

disproportion lack of fit between two objects, e.g. referring to the relationship in which the fetal head is too large to pass through the maternal pelvis.

disseminated intravascular coagulation (DIC) a condition in which there is widespread consumption of clotting factors and failure of haemostasis.

distal situated furthest from point of attachment or origin, as of a limb or bone. The opposite of distal is proximal.

distress suffering; exhaustion; in danger; a level of stress/stimulation considered to be detrimental to health.

diuresis increased secretion of urine.

diurnal occurring in the daytime.

dizygotic twins two babies in the same pregnancy developed from two ova released simultaneously.

DNA abbreviation for deoxyribonucleic acid. The substance found in the chromosomes of nucleus which carries coded genetic information and is capable of reproduction.

DNA testing examination of deoxyribonucleic acid (DNA). Can detect inherited disease carriers and determine paternity.

Döderlein's bacillus (*Lactobacillus acidophilus*) a gram-positive bacillus which is a normal inhabitant of the vagina. These bacilli digest glucose to form lactic acid which protects against infection.

dolichocephalic having a relatively long head.

domestic violence (DV) any incidence of controlling, coercive, threatening behaviour, violence or abuse between those who are, or have been, intimate partners or family members regardless of gender or sexuality. The abuse can encompass, but is not limited to: psychological, physical, sexual, financial or emotional (also referred to as intimate partner violence).

dominance expression of control.

dominant gene term applied to the one gene out of two genes which will shape the future individual. The capacity of one gene to exert control or express its characteristic trait in the presence of a similar gene.

dominant inheritance a hereditary pattern in which one gene of a pair overrules the characteristic expression of the other.

donor one who gives blood or tissue to another.

donor insemination the use of sperm from a donor in order to attempt conception.

doppler ultrasound scanning a procedure used to assess the flow of blood through vessels; used to visualise the flow of fetal blood through the umbilical vessels.

dorsal referring to the posterior part of an organ.

dose the measured quantity of a medicine to be given at any one time.

double-blind trial a research study in which an intervention is administered to one proportion of the sample and a placebo to the other but neither the subjects nor the administrators know which group is receiving active intervention, thereby avoiding subjectivity and removing potential bias.

double uterus (SYNONYM uterus didelphys) congenital condition where the paramesonephric ducts in the uterus did not unite during embryonic development, leading to a double uterus with double cervix and double vagina.

douche washing, lavage, using a stream of water, usually applied to the genitals.

doula a lay person or birth attendant who provides non-clinical support and advocacy to a woman throughout labour. Doulas may also provide postnatal support.

Down syndrome (SYNONYM trisomy 21) a congenital defect of chromosome resulting in variable levels of disability. An extra chromosome 21 is present.

droplet infection an infection transmitted from one individual to another through the air. It is commonly spread due to sneezing or coughing.

drug a chemical compound given to change the responses of the body to its environment; substance used for medical purposes.

drug abuse the effect of substances being introduced into the body other than for therapeutic use; overuse of a drug for enhanced stimulant, hallucinogenic or other non-therapeutic effect that results in addiction.

drug addiction the inability of an individual to function without certain substances in their blood.

drug concentration the measurable amount of a substance in the blood when tested to determine uptake and to guide further therapeutic administration.

drug-induced teratogenesis a congenital abnormality resulting from the absorption of a certain substance which alters genetic coding and cellular development in the fetus.

drug resistance the lack of sensitivity or expected response to a therapeutic preparation; the ability of microorganisms to withstand the effect of an antibiotic substance.

drug tolerance the gradually acquired ability to resist the effect of a drug; acquired insensitivity; the requirement to increase the dose of a drug regularly to maintain the same effect.

Dubowitz score an assessment devised for determining gestational age of infants based on several physical and behavioural characteristics.

Duchenne's muscular dystrophy an eventually fatal disorder that is characterised by rapidly progressive muscle weakness and atrophy of muscle tissue.

duct a tube conveying secretions away from their source.

ductus arteriosus a bypass blood vessel that shunts blood between the left pulmonary artery and the aorta in fetal life; it normally closes at birth.

ductus venosus a venous channel in the fetus, the umbilical vein passing through the liver and joining into the inferior vena cava.

Duffy blood group a blood group consisting mainly of the antigens fy(a) and fy(b).

duodenum the first part of the small intestine.

duplex having two parts.

dura mater toughened fibromembranous lining of the skull, forming the outermost covering of the brain tissue and spinal cord.

dural tap a complication of the epidural procedure in which cerebrospinal fluid leaks. Severe headache occurs and lasts several days.

duty of care the requirement of a professionally trained person to behave in a prescribed manner.

dwarfism short stature caused by genetic alteration, endocrine conditions or chronic disease.

dys- prefix meaning disordered, abnormal, difficult or painful.

dysfunctional uterine bleeding (DUB) bleeding from the uterus not associated with pregnancy, tumour or menstruation.

dyskaryosis irregularity in nuclear shape or number.

dyslexia a learning disability that may involve variations in reading and writing proficiency.

dysmaturity the failure of an organism or fetus to achieve expected development. This term may be applied to a fetus that is small for gestational age or one that is large for gestational age but whose behaviour is immature.

dysmenorrhoea difficult or painful menstruation.

dysmorphia deformity.

dyspareunia difficult or painful coitus.

dyspnoea difficult or laboured breathing.

dystocia difficult or problematic labour. In *shoulder dystocia*, the head emerges but the shoulders fail to be born easily.

dysuria difficult or painful urination.

Ee

E, e symbol used to denote Rh blood types, others being C, c and D, d.

external anal sphincter (EAS) outer sphincter of striated muscle controlling the closure of the anus. Can sustain damage during birth.

E. coli (*Escherichia coli*) a gram-negative bacterium which normally inhabits the intestine. Outside of the intestinal tract it causes infection.

e-cigarette a device that allows a person to inhale nicotine in a vapour, rather than smoke (*see also* vaping).

early cord clamping umbilical cord clamping undertaken within 1 minute after birth.

early neonatal death death of a live-born baby within 7 days of birth.

early onset Group B streptococcal disease neonatal infection that occurs within the first 7 days of life. Most commonly within 72 hours of birth (*see* Group B streptococcal bacteria).

Ebstein's anomaly a congenital heart condition in which the tricuspid valve is located deep into the right ventricle creating obstruction to filling and other symptoms including heart failure.

ecchymosis bruising caused by leakage of blood into the subcutaneous tissue.

ECG (electrocardiogram) a measurement of the electrical activity in the heart during contraction which can be recorded in graphic form.

echoencephalography pulsed echo or ultrasound used to examine the intracranial structures.

eclampsia seizure or convulsion usually associated with pre-eclampsia.

ECMO *see* extracorporeal membrane oxygenation.

ecto- combining form meaning outside or out of place, as in *ectopic pregnancy*.

ectoderm the outermost of the three primary germinal layers of the embryo.

-ectomy combining form meaning surgical cutting away of tissue.

ectopic not in the normal position.

ectopic pregnancy pregnancy developing outside the uterine cavity, usually in the fallopian tube but sometimes in the abdominal cavity. The pregnancy outgrows the blood supply by 10 weeks and erodes blood vessels which bleed creating a maternity emergency.

ectro- prefix meaning miscarriage, congenital absence.

ectrodactyly a congenital condition in which there is absence of one or more fingers or toes or parts of them.

ectromelia condition where one or more long bones of one or more limbs do not grow normally and are hypoplastic.

ectropion eversion of a part, e.g. the eyelid or cervix.

ectrosyndactyly a condition in which some of the digits are missing and those that remain are webbed, so that they are more or less attached.

eczema an inflammatory condition of the skin characterised by a combination of itching, redness, scaling and production of exudate. Usually congenital but may be set off by artificial feeding in sensitive babies.

Edward's syndrome (trisomy 18) a genetic condition due to the presence of an extra chromosome (18). People with the syndrome usually have intellectual disability and specific physical signs such as skull abnormalities, micrognathia, blepharoptosis, low-set ears, corneal opacities, deafness, webbed neck, short digits, ventricular septal defects, Meckel's diverticulum.

EEG *see* electroencephalogram.

effacement loss of form of the uterine cervix during labour (*see* Fig. 29).

efferent carrying or conducting away from centre to peripheries.

effusion the pouring out of any fluid into surrounding tissue or cavity.

egg collection the event in IVF treatment where the woman's eggs are collected for later fertilisation.

ejaculation 1. sudden explosion or emission. 2. release of semen.

elasticity the characteristic of being able to stretch and return to original shape. *Elastic stockings* are knee-high or thigh-high self-retaining stockings applied before surgery, e.g. caesarean section, to prevent pooling of blood in the legs thereby reducing the risk of thrombosis occurring.

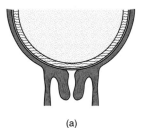
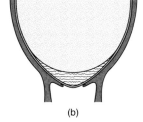

(a)   (b)

Figure 29
Effacement of cervix

elective done by choice; *elective surgery* is planned surgery which is neither urgent nor mandatory.

elective caesarean section caesarean section done at a time and date of choice before the onset of labour.

electrocardiogram (ECG) a graphical record of electrical impulses emitted by the heart during a cardiac cycle.

electrode a conductor transmitting an electrical wave from its source to another medium or instrument. Fetal scalp electrodes are attached to the fetal scalp and record the heart activity on a printout.

electroencephalogram (EEG) a graphic record of electrical waves emitted by the cerebral cortex.

electrolyte a substance which in solution is capable of conducting electrical current.

electrolyte balance the balance between the salts, sodium, potassium and chlorides in bodily fluids.

electrolyte solution a fluid that is capable of conducting an electric current.

electronic fetal monitor (EFM) an electronic method of recording fetal heart activity using a cardiotocograph. Uterine activity is recorded at the same time.

elimination the process of expelling the waste products of the body.

embolism the occlusion of a blood vessel by particulate, clots, air, amniotic fluid or foreign body which travels from another part of the body, e.g. *pulmonary embolism*.

embolus a foreign body, air, gas, tumour, liquor or clot of blood which moves around the circulation.

embryectomy surgical removal of an extrauterine embryo, as is done as a result of an ectopic pregnancy.

embryo the early stage of development—from fertilisation to the end of the 8th week of gestation (*see* Fig. 30).

embryo transfer where the embryo is transferred back to the woman's uterus via a fine catheter as part of IVF treatment.

embryology the scientific study of early human development.

embryonal carcinoma a cancer of embryonic cells.

embryonic abortion termination of a pregnancy before the 12th week of gestation.

embryonic disc the three-layer plate of cells from which the embryo develops in the 2nd week of pregnancy.

embryonic stage the stage of pregnancy from the end of the germinal stage on 10th day until the end of the 8th week.

embryotomy intentional destruction of an embryo in utero to facilitate removal when natural delivery is impossible.

emergency sudden development of pathological condition which requires immediate medical attention.

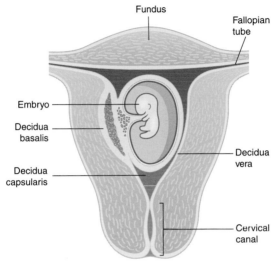

Figure 30
Embryo

emesis the act of vomiting.
eminence a projection, prominent part of a bone.
emmenagogue an agent or measure that induces menstruation.
emollient a substance which softens tissue or soothes an inflammation.
emotion psychologic strong feelings often accompanied by outward expression of mood change.
emotional deprivation absence of affection, regard, interest or encouragement of one person towards another, usually a parent for a child.
empathy ability to understand the feelings or emotions of another person.
empowerment the process by which women are enabled to make their own decisions and choices, based on all available knowledge and without being influenced by others, and feel strong in their own decisions.
empty follicle syndrome a condition in which there are no oocytes in a Graafian follicle.

encephalin (enkephalin) one of two naturally occurring substances in the brain which are neurotransmitters and have an opiate-like effect, suppressing the sensation of pain.

encephalitis inflammation of the brain tissue.

encephalocele hernia of the brain tissue through a congenital or traumatic opening in the skull.

endemic describes an infectious disease which is always present to a lesser or greater degree in a particular locality.

endo- combining form meaning within or inner.

endocervical pertaining to the endocervix.

endocervicitis inflammation of the epithelium and glands within the cervix.

endocervix the glandular mucous membrane lining the uterine cervix.

endocrine system glands which secrete their produce, mainly hormones, directly into the bloodstream.

endoderm the innermost of the three layers forming the embryonic disc which will form the cavities, passages and internal organs of the developing fetus.

endogenous produced from within (*compare* exogenous).

endometrial referring to the inner layer or mucous membrane lining the cavity of the uterus.

endometrial hyperplasia an overgrowth of the endometrial lining resulting from oestrogen stimulation without the controlling effect of progesterone.

endometrial polyp an overgrowth of endometrium which has formed on a stalk; it may protrude through the cervix. Usually benign but may cause abnormal bleeding.

endometriosis presence of functional endometrial tissue in abnormal locations, outside the uterus.

endometrium the mucous membrane lining the inside of the body of the uterine cavity.

endorphins a number of different neuropeptides which act on the central nervous system and reduce the sensation of pain.

endotoxins poisonous substances released from the cell walls of microorganisms. *Endotoxic shock* is a sudden physical collapse associated with septicaemia.

endotracheal tube a plastic tube that is inserted into the nose or mouth and down into the trachea to maintain the patient's airway during anaesthesia. Material or fluid is prevented from entering the lungs beside the tube using a cuff that is inflated once the tube is inserted in the correct spot.

enema introduction of fluid into the rectum to clear the contents.

engagement entry of the presenting part of the fetus

into the true pelvis such that the widest part is below the brim.

engorgement a state of being overfilled. Engorgement of the breasts may occur as milk 'comes in' during lactation.

ensiform cartilage (xiphoid process) small extension of cartilage at the lower part of the sternum, usually ossified in adults.

enteric referring to the intestines.

enteritis inflammation of the intestinal mucosa.

entoderm the innermost of the three primary germ layers of the inner cell mass which will become the internal organs of the fetus.

Entonox® an analgesic preparation consisting of premixed gases—50% nitrous oxide and 50% oxygen. Inhaled during labour contractions to dull the pain sensation.

enuresis involuntary urination, which may be caused by a variety of factors. Bedwetting.

environmental health the totality of the various substances, gases, forces and attitudes in and about a community which affect the health of members of that community.

enzyme a substance capable of breaking down another substance by a chemical reaction.

eosin a red acid dye used in histopathology for staining bacteria or cells.

eosinophil a white granulocytic cell whose granules stain red with eosin.

epicanthus skin fold of the upper eyelid. More common in some ethnic backgrounds and sometimes indicates the presence of a congenital anomaly.

epidemic an outbreak of a specific disease extending throughout a local community.

epidemiology branch of science concerned with examining factors that determine and influence frequency and distribution of disease, injury and other health-related events.

epidermal naevus (naevus verrucous) a brown, warty lesion on the discoloured skin of the newborn caused by an overgrowth of epidermis.

epidermis the top or superficial layer of the skin.

epidermolysis bullosa a hereditary skin condition characterised by widespread development of vesicles on contact, without the occurrence of trauma.

epididymis the tightly coiled single duct into which spermatozoa are deposited and reach complete maturation before passing into the vas deferens.

epidural situated over the dura mater.

epidural analgesia introduction of an anaesthetic agent into the epidural space resulting in blocking of pain sensation.

epidural blood patch treatment employed in the management of a dural puncture sustained during epidural catheterisation. A small volume of the woman's blood is injected into the dural space; the clot which forms seals the breach and prevents further leakage of cerebrospinal fluid.

epigastric pertaining to the upper middle section of the abdomen.

epigastric pain pain in the upper area of the abdomen.

epigastric region the upper middle part of the abdomen.

epigenetics the study of changes in organisms caused by modification of gene expression as opposed to changes in the genetic code or DNA.

epilepsy recurring episodes of neurological malfunction including motor and sensory lapses or convulsive seizures and unconsciousness.

epinephrine *see* adrenaline.

episiorrhaphy repair of an episiotomy.

episiotomy cut made into the perineum/pelvic floor during childbirth to enlarge the vaginal orifice.

epispadias a congenital defect in which the urethral canal opens on the underside of the penis.

epistaxis nosebleed.

epithelium a tissue compound identified by shape and function lining all inner body surfaces.

epoprostenol (prostacyclin) (PG1) one of the prostaglandin hormones. It is metabolised in vascular walls and inhibits platelet aggregation.

Epstein's pearls small white spots found on both sides of the hard palate in the mouth of a newborn baby.

Erb's palsy upper brachial plexus nerve damage resulting in paralysis of the upper arm.

erectile capable of becoming firm or dilated.

erectile tissue spongy tissue which, as a result of venous engorgement, becomes rigid and enlarged (*see* Fig. 31). The penis and the nipple both contain erectile tissue.

ergot a fungus developed on rye, the alkaloids of which are used in the manufacture of oxytocins.

erosion of the cervix destruction of superficial squamous epithelium and exposure of columnar epithelial cells of the endocervix.

erythema patchy redness of the skin.

erythema neonatorum patchy redness of variable size and shape on the body of a neonate. May be caused by heat, irritants or drugs but usually disappears after several days.

erythroblast an immature erythrocyte in which a nucleus is present.

erythroblastosis fetalis a haemolytic anaemia in the

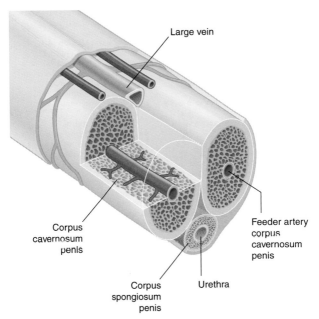

Figure 31
Erectile tissue

neonate resulting from maternal–fetal blood group incompatibility. The mother may form antibodies to the fetus's foreign antigen where it is of a differing Rh factor or ABO blood group.

erythrocyte a mature non-nucleated red blood cell able to transport oxygen around the body.

erythropoiesis the process by which red blood cells are formed.

Escherichia coli *see E.coli.*

essential hypertension high blood pressure that has no identifiable cause.

estimated date of birth (EDB) a projected guess of the date on which the baby will be born. It is estimated using

Nägele's rule, and calculations may be adjusted to take into account personal factors such as menstrual history and ultrasound measurements early in pregnancy.

estimated date of delivery (EDD) *see* estimated date of birth.

estradiol, estriol *see* oestrogen.

estrone an oestrogen which can be isolated in the urine during pregnancy.

ethnic group a social group with shared values, beliefs, history and sometimes religion.

ethnography the study of an aspect of the life of a single culture, race or group within society.

eugenics branch of science concerned with gene selection and improvement of stock.

euphoria an extreme feeling of physical and mental wellbeing, often not based in reality.

eustachian tube the narrow tube which connects the tympanum (middle ear) with the naso-pharynx.

eutocia normal childbirth and labour.

evacuation emptying of the contents of, e.g. uterus or bowel.

evaluate assess the value or worth of something, e.g. research results, care management.

evidence statement or facts used as proof.

ex- combining form meaning outside, out of.

exacerbation an increase in the severity of a disease; making worse.

exchange transfusion a methodical and gradual withdrawal of almost all of a person's volume of blood and replacement with that provided by a donor. Can be done for neonates with severe jaundice and Rh incompatibility.

excision the cutting away of a part of an organ or tissue.

excreta waste materials which have been removed from the body.

exercise physical activity or training to sustain or improve health.

exogenous originating from an external source (*compare* endogenous).

exomphalos a herniation of abdominal content into the umbilicus. It may or may not be covered with skin.

experiment an investigation in which one or more factors in a situation may be examined, altered and the effects studied; procedures used for testing a hypothesis.

expert witness a person with a great deal of experience and knowledge in a particular area who is able to testify or give evidence in a court of law.

expertise special skill in or knowledge of a particular area.

expression 1. pressing out. 2. pressure on the uterus to facilitate the expulsion of the placenta.

expulsion the act of forcing out, e.g. a fetus from the uterus.

expulsive stage of labour the period in labour after full dilation of the cervix during which the mother feels an overwhelming urge to use her abdominal muscles to push the fetus through the birth canal.

exsanguinate to empty of blood. This can happen to a fetus if the umbilical cord ruptures.

extended family the cousins, aunts, uncles, grandparents and significant others in a tightly knit group living in a large household or in close proximity to each other.

extension an action by which a flexed part is straightened out, e.g. the fetal head.

external ballottement bimanual examination in which an organ is tapped in an attempt to displace its contents which rebound and settle against the examiner's hand.

external fertilisation the sperm and ovum fuse outside the body, e.g. in a laboratory, as in in vitro fertilisation (IVF).

external os uteri the opening in the cervix nearest the outside.

external version transabdominal manipulation of the fetus by which the lie or presentation is altered.

extracorporeal membrane oxygenation supportive strategy that is also called a life support machine whereby oxygenation of blood takes place outside the body. Also known as extracorporeal life support (ECLS).

extrauterine outside the uterine cavity.

extrauterine pregnancy one that occurs outside of the uterus, as in an ectopic or an abdominal pregnancy.

extravasation leakage of body fluids out of the appropriate place or into surrounding tissues.

extrinsic of external origin.

extrophy malformation of an organ.

extubation removal of a tube used in intubation.

exudates fluids such as sweat or protein-rich substances and cells which leak out of the body through pores or pass through vessel walls into adjacent tissue.

Ff

F abbreviation for Fahrenheit, a scale of temperature measurement in which water freezes at 32°F and boiling point is 212°F.

face anterior part of the head extending from the forehead to chin. In the fetus it is the area between the supraorbital ridges and the mentum.

face presentation an extended cephalic presentation of the fetus. The chin is extended. The face will be felt on vaginal examination. The baby's face is born facing upwards towards the mother's face rather than facing backwards towards her spine, as in the birth of an anteriorly positioned baby (*see* Fig. 32).

face-to-pubes birth occurs with a cephalic presentation, usually when the head is not fully flexed and has passed through the pelvis in an occipitoposterior position. As

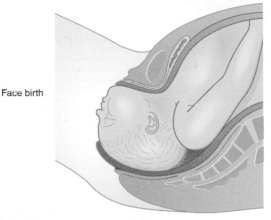

Face birth

Figure 32
Face presentation at birth

crowning occurs the brow will be seen under the symphysis pubis. The occipit sweeps the perineum as it is born by flexion. It will probably be born before the face has completely emerged from under the symphysis pubis.

facial palsy damage to the 7th cranial nerve resulting in partial or total weakness of the muscles of expression. Occasionally occurs as a result of a forceps delivery.

facilitator a person who enables or encourages another person to explore or discover information necessary to fulfil their needs.

factor a substance which promotes or enables a particular physiological function.

factors I, II, III, IV, V, VI, VII, VIII, IX, X, XI, XII, XIII names given to substances which enable blood to clot.

faeces food residue expelled as waste material from the bowels.

failed forceps unsuccessful attempt at birth of the fetal head using obstetric forceps. An emergency caesarean section may be required.

failure to thrive *see* faltering growth.

faint sudden lapse of consciousness resulting from a fall in blood pressure and cerebral hypoxia.

fallopian tubes the two oviducts or uterine tubes extending from the cornua and branching out to surround the ovary.

Fallot's tetralogy four congenital heart defects occurring together.

false labour discomfort or pain caused by uterine contractions but not resulting in cervical dilation. Use of the term false is often not helpful for women to hear.

false negative an incorrect diagnostic result indicating the absence of a pathological state when a disease is actually present.

false pelvis the region of the pelvis above the iliopectineal line.

false positive an incorrect diagnostic result suggesting that there is an abnormality when there is not.

false pregnancy *see* pseudocyesis.

faltering growth deficit in the expected development of the infant. The neonate does not gain weight or meet the expected milestones. Previously called failure to thrive. Previously called failure to thrive.

falx a sickle-shaped structure.

falx cerebelli the sickle-shaped membrane of dura mater attached to the occipital bone and located between the two cerebral hemispheres.

falx cerebri the sickle-shaped, doublefold dura mater separating the two cerebral hemispheres.

familial pertaining to or occurring among family members.

family a group of people descended from a common

ancestor; parents and children.

family planning premeditated measures adopted for preventing, limiting or timing the spacing of the birth of children.

Farber test microscopic examination of the meconium to detect lanugo, cells and ingested substances, the absence of which suggests intestinal obstruction.

fascia the fibrous sheath of connective tissue between muscles or loosely applied around organs, nerves and blood vessels.

fasting abstaining from food (but not water).

fatal resulting in death.

fear emotion based on anxiety and acute sense of alarm associated with an event or object.

febrile characterised by fever.

fecundation the process of fertilisation.

fecundity the ability to procreate.

feed to provide with nutrition; to give food to an infant by breast, bottle, tube or other means.

female circumcision, female genital mutilation excision of various parts of the female genitalia (labia minora, clitoris and labia majora) for non-therapeutic reasons. This practice is illegal in many countries.

female pseudohermaphrodite congenital abnormality of the external genitalia where the gender cannot be determined by examination of the external characteristics but ovaries are present.

feminism the promotion of women's rights to be equal to those of men.

femoral pertaining to the femur or thigh bone.

fenestrated possessing a window-like opening or *fenestra*.

Ferguson's reflex the uncontrollable desire to bear down and aid expulsion of the fetus, triggered by pressure from the presenting part stimulating nerves in the pelvic floor.

fern test the pattern created by dried crystallised cervical mucus on a glass slide post ovulation. Indicative of the presence of an oestrogen surge.

ferritin an iron–protein complex. A form of iron stored in tissues.

fertile able to produce offspring.

fertile period the days in the menstrual cycle after ovulation during which a pregnancy is likely to occur.

fertilisation the union of male and female gametes (*see* Fig. 33).

fertility rate the number of births per 1000 women.

fetal pertaining to the fetus or unborn baby.

fetal alcohol spectrum disorder (FASD) a spectrum of conditions caused by exposure to alcohol by the unborn baby. The features of

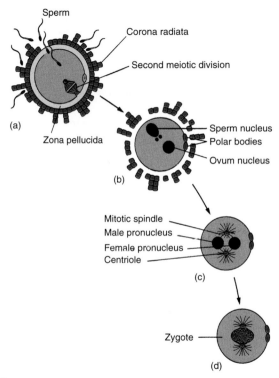

Figure 33
Fertilisation

the condition may be physical, developmental and/or neurobehavioural.

fetal blood sampling procedure performed in labour, whereby a small sample of blood is obtained from the scalp of the baby for estimation of pH, lactate and other parameters as a means of determining fetal wellbeing (*see* Fig. 34).

fetal bradycardia a fetal heart rate of less than 110 bpm at term (normal 110–160 bpm).

fetal circulation the cardiovascular network in the fetus including the placenta and umbilical cord (*see* Fig. 35).

fetal death death of the baby in utero before the onset of labour. Typically defined as after 20 weeks' gestation.

fetal haemoglobin (HbF) the dominant haemoglobin in intrauterine life, though small quantities continue to be produced throughout life. It is highly receptive to oxygen but is fragile and therefore short-lived.

fetal heart rate (FHR) the number of times the fetal heart beats in 1 minute— normal range is between 110 and 160 beats per minute.

fetal heart sounds the sound of the fetal heart beat which can be auscultated and counted.

fetal hypoxia a state of reduced delivery of oxygen to the baby.

fetal movements movements made by the baby in utero. These are present from the beginning of pregnancy and are usually felt by the woman from the 16th to 19th week of gestation.

fetal skull the entire bony structure of the fetal head including the three regions of face, vault and base.

feticide the destruction or killing of a fetus in utero.

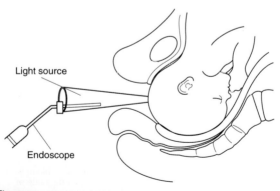

Light source

Endoscope

Figure 34
Fetal blood sampling

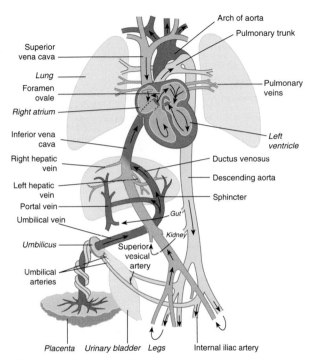

Figure 35
Fetal circulation

---

fetology the study of the fetus in utero.

fetoplacental referring to the fetus and placenta to which it is attached as one unit/ organism.

fetoscopy transabdominal introduction of an instrument into the uterine cavity for visual inspection of the fetus.

fetus (SYNONYM the baby) term applied to mammalian

offspring from the beginning of the 9th week after fertilisation until birth.

fetus papyraceous one of twin fetuses that has died early in pregnancy and has been flattened by the survivor to resemble a paper cutout.

fetus sanguinolentis a fetus that has died and started to decompose and is born with dark blood patches visible beneath the skin.

fever a rise in body temperature above normal limits.

fibrin an insoluble protein formed by the interaction of thrombin and fibrinogen during clot formation.

fibrinogen the soluble protein precursor of fibrin present in blood plasma.

fibrinolysin the enzyme in the blood which dissolves fibrin.

fibroid a dense mass of adherent fibrous tissue. A benign tumour found within the muscle of the uterus.

fibromyoma a benign tumour of uterine muscle; a fibroid.

fibromyomectomy surgical removal of a fibroid.

fight or flight reaction a state of heightened preparedness for sudden activity resulting from a surge of adrenaline (epinephrine) in the circulation as a consequence of great stress. Larger amounts of energy become available and peripheral circulation is depleted. It is counterproductive in labour.

filter a porous membrane-like structure which permits selective passage of some compounds while restricting the passage of others.

filtrate the solution that has passed through a filter.

fimbria 1. a fringe. 2. the fringe-like dilated extremity of the fallopian tube.

fimbria ovarica the fringe or fringe-like end of the fallopian tube which is nearest to the ovary.

first-degree perineal tear laceration of the perineum involving only the skin or fourchette.

first stage of labour the interval from the onset of active labour to complete dilation of the cervix.

fission 1. cleavage or splitting. 2. a method of asexual reproduction.

fissure 1. groove or cleft normally occurring in the body. 2. ulceration or crack in the skin.

fistula abnormal communication between two surfaces or organs.

fit a convulsion or seizure.

flaccid relaxed or without tone; soft, flabby, limp.

flagellum (PLURAL flagella) thin, whip-like process contained in cytoplasm, movement of which enables propulsion in certain bacteria and sperm cells.

flank the side abdominal region between the ribs and hip.

flaring of nostrils dilation of the nares (nostrils) to aid respiratory effort where breathing is difficult, e.g. in respiratory distress syndrome in a preterm neonate.

flat pelvis (SYNONYM platypelloid pelvis) a pelvis with reduced anteroposterior and increased transverse diameters and a shallow cavity.

flatulence an excess of gas in the stomach or intestines.

fleshy mole *see* carneous mole.

flexion the state of being bent. The normal attitude or position of the fetal head in relation to its body in utero.

flooding term used to describe heavy menstrual blood flow.

flora bacteria found in the large intestine which enable the body to manufacture essential vitamins such as vitamin K and protect against invasion by pathological organisms.

fluid balance the maintenance of optimal water content for physiological function by regulating intake and output.

fluid overload excessive accumulation of fluid within the body as a result of over-transfusion of intravenous solutions.

fluid thrill a clinical sign indicative of polyhydramnios. A ripple or wave effect can be seen over the abdomen when one side is tapped.

folate a general term used to describe a large group of compounds.

Foley catheter a balloon-tipped retainable urinary catheter.

folic acid a vitamin of the B complex group found in green leafy vegetables, liver and yeast; essential to the development of healthy erythrocytes.

follicle a small secretory sac or cavity.

follicle stimulating hormone (FSH) pituitary hormone which stimulates growth and maturation of ovarian follicles or spermatogenesis in the testes.

follicular phase the early period of the menstrual cycle during which the Graafian follicle is growing and ripening.

fontanelle a membranous space between the cranial bones in the baby (*see* Fig. 36).

footling presentation a variation of the breech presentation in which one foot is presenting in front of the buttocks.

foramen an opening or perforation, especially in a bone.

foramen magnum the spinal cord passes this large opening at the base of the skull.

foramen ovale oval window; a physiological opening in the septum of the heart through which blood is shunted from the right to left atrium in fetal life, bypassing the lungs.

forceps a two-bladed surgical instrument used to grasp or compress body tissues or objects.

forceps-assisted birth an assisted birth in which

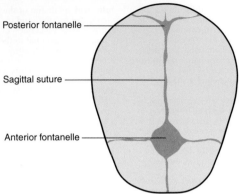

Figure 36
Fontanelle

extraction of the baby is
enabled after the application
of the forceps to the head
and traction is applied (*see*
Fig. 37).

forceps rotation use of
Kielland's rotational forceps
which have long handles and
flat or less-defined curvatures
of the blade to correct
malposition of the fetal
head.

foremilk the first milk drawn
at each breastfeed.

foreskin (SYNONYM prepuce)
the skin covering the glans
penis.

forewaters the pool of
amniotic fluid lying in front
of the presenting part and
separated from the main
volume (*see* Fig. 38).

formaldehyde a powerful
disinfectant.

formula 1. rules expressed
in symbols. 2. laboratory-
prepared recipe of modified
cows' milk or other
substitutes for feeding
infants.

fornication 1. sexual
intercourse. 2. historically,
sexual intercourse outside
marriage.

fornix 1. a cul-de-sac or
arch-shaped structure. 2. the
recessed arched vault of the
vagina between the cervix
and the vaginal walls (*see*
Fig. 39).

fossa a depression or hollow.

fourchette a fold of skin at the
posterior aspect of the labia
minora.

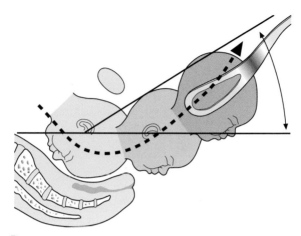

Figure 37
Forceps-assisted birth

fracture break of a bone or cartilage.

fracture of the clavicle a break in the long bone lying between the shoulder girdle and the sternum. It may be deliberately broken (cleidotomy) to release the baby's shoulder in cases of shoulder dystocia.

fracture of the skull a break in one of the bones of the skull. May occur following a forceps delivery.

frank extended breech the fetus is presenting with the buttocks over the cervical os, the thighs are flexed and the legs are extended

to lie alongside the shoulders.

frenulum a small fold of mucous membrane acting as a restraining ligament.

frenulum of the tongue the membranous cord which attaches the tongue to the floor of the mouth.

friable easily broken or torn, crumbly.

Friedman's curve a curved line on preprinted partograms which indicates the expected progress of labour based on research undertaken by Friedman in the 1950s.

frigid historical term used to describe a woman who does

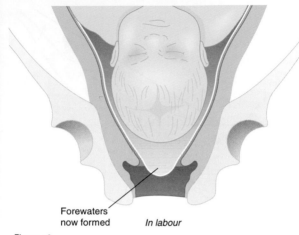

Forewaters
now formed   *In labour*

Figure 38
Forewaters

not experience sexual arousal
or enjoy sexual intercourse.
frontal pertaining to the
anterior aspect of the body or
the forehead.
FSH *see* follicle stimulating
hormone.
full term a term used to
describe a woman who has
reached 37 completed weeks
of pregnancy or beyond.
fulminating sudden, severe
and rapid in onset or
progression.
fulminating pre-eclampsia
condition in which a
woman with pre-eclampsia is
at risk of experiencing a
seizure.

fundal referring to the fundus,
or top of the uterus.
fundal force (fundal pressure)
the application of force to the
top of the uterus to aid the
birth of the infant in the
second stage of labour or the
placenta in the third stage.
Not generally considered safe
in current practice, except in
emergency situations.
fundal height estimation of the
gestational age by measuring
the distance from the top of
the uterus to the symphysis
pubis.
fundal placenta a placenta
normally located in the top or
fundus of the uterus.

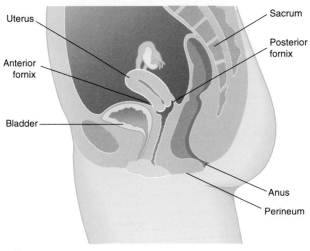

Figure 39
Fornix

---

fundus the base of an organ or
the part furthest removed
from the opening.
fungal infection pathogenic
condition caused by a fungus
or yeast.
funic referring to the umbilical
cord (funis).
funic souffle a soft blowing
murmur emitted from the
umbilical cord and usually

synchronous with the beating
of the fetal heart.
funnel pelvis a pelvis in which
there is progressive reduction
of the diameters from the
brim to outlet.
fusion joining together, e.g. of
organs, cavities or tubes.
Dividing walls are removed
by ingestion by enzymes.

Gg

g (gm) abbreviation for gram.

G6PD *see* glucose-6-phosphate dehydrogenase.

gag 1. to retch. 2. an instrument used to prevent closure of the jaw.

gag reflex constriction of the pharyngeal muscle in response to stimulation of the soft palate; the tongue is pulled back to protect the airway.

gait a manner of walking or carrying one's body.

galactagogue an agent that increases the secretion of milk.

galacto-, galact- combining form denoting milk.

galactorrhoea lactation not associated with childbirth.

galactosaemia inability to convert galactose to glucose. Caused by an inborn error of metabolism in which the galactose-splitting enzyme galactose-1-phosphate uridyl transferase is either deficient or absent.

galactose a monosaccharide produced after the metabolism of lactose.

galactosis secretion of milk by the mammary glands.

Galant reflex induced sideways flexion of the neonate's hips in the direction of contact when the lower back is stroked.

Galen's vein (vein of Galen) the large cerebral vein which drains blood from the midbrain. During abnormal moulding or a difficult birth it may rupture causing severe intracranial haemorrhage.

gall bile.

gall bladder a hollow, pear-shaped structure situated on the undersurface of the liver in which bile is stored and concentrated.

gamete the reproductive cells capable of fertilisation.

gamete intrafallopian transfer (GIFT) ovum and sperm are collected, prepared, then returned together to the fallopian tube for fertilisation to occur.

gametocyte a cell which has the potential to become a sperm or ovum.

gametogenesis the process of formation and development of gametes.

gametophyte a stage in the process of gamete development at which the nuclei are haploid.

gamma globulin a group of immunoglobulins (A, D, E, G and M) with specific antibody activity.

ganglion a body of nerve cells from which other fibres or tendrils extend.

gangrene tissue death and necrosis due to failure or interruption of blood supply.

Gardnerella vaginalis a rod-shaped gram-negative bacterium normally found in the vagina. *Gardnerella vaginalis vaginitis* is the inflammation and symptoms resulting from bacterial infection with *Gardnerella*; thought to be transmitted sexually.

Gardasil (SYNONYM Gardasil, Silgard, recombinant human papillomavirus vaccine) vaccine to prevent infection by specific strains of human papillomavirus (HPV) (types 6, 11, 16 and 18). These strains are responsible for cervical cancers and most HPV-induced anal, vulvar, vaginal and penile cancer cases.

gas matter in vaporous state, being neither solid nor liquid.

Gaskin manoeuvre the hands and knees position that women may choose to adopt in labour and during birth (*see* Fig. 40). It is specifically useful to reduce shoulder dystocia.

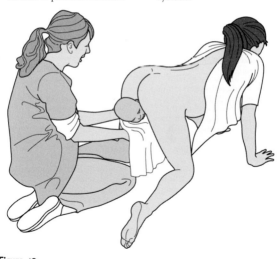

Figure 40
Gaskin manoeuvre
Illustration by Alan Laver

gastric juices secretions of the glands in the stomach; these are strongly acidic and digest food.

gastric lavage washing out of the stomach.

gastric tube feeding (SYNONYM nasogastric feeding/orogastric feeding) introduction of food into the stomach via a tube. A method often employed in the care of premature or sick babies.

gastro- combining form meaning pertaining to the stomach.

gastroenteritis inflammation of the stomach and intestinal mucosa; usually accompanied by vomiting and diarrhoea.

gastroschisis a congenital fissure of the abdominal wall.

gastrostomy the creation of an opening into the stomach.

gate control theory of pain suggests there is selection or competition as to which impulses will travel up the spine and be received in the brain, e.g. sensations such as electricity across the skin or pain from contraction compete. When transcutaneous electrical nerve stimulation (TENS) is used, electricity, rather than pain, passes up the spinal nerves.

GBS *see* Group B streptococcal bacteria.

GBV *see* gender-based violence.

gel a thick substance with a high concentration of water used as a lubricant or to deliver medicine.

gemellology the scientific study of twins and twinning.

gender the classification of people as female or male.

gender-based violence (GBV) harmful acts directed at an individual based on their gender. Commonly refers to violence towards girls and women and includes physical, sexual or mental harm or suffering. *See also* GBV.

gender identity an inner sense of oneself as man, woman, masculine, feminine, neither, both or moving around freely between or outside of the gender binary.

gender pronouns how a person chooses to publicly express their gender identity through the use of a pronoun. Includes 'she' or 'he' and gender-neutral pronouns such as 'they', 'their', 'ze' and 'hir'.

gene a unit of hereditary factor capable of transmitting specific genetic code and occupying a defined position on a chromosome.

gene pool the total number of genetic traits available within a population.

general anaesthesia a drug-induced medical state in which there is combined loss of sensation and consciousness.

general practitioner (GP) a doctor engaged in primary practice within the community.

generation all people considered to be within a specific age band; the time between the birth of an individual and the birth of his/her offspring.

generic drugs refers to the chemical make-up of a drug rather than the brand name.

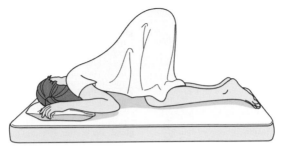

Figure 41
Genupectoral position
Illustration by Alan Laver

genetic pertaining to genes; having reference to the origin of development.

genetic carrier a person who carries a 'faulty' gene which can be passed on to his or her children but who displays no signs of it or of ill health.

genetic counselling detailed explanation of the risks of transmitting a hereditary condition to one's children and presentation of options or reproductive alternatives.

genetic engineering manipulation of genetic characteristics by removal or insertion of foreign gene materials.

genetic screening DNA analysis of blood samples to determine which characteristic an offspring is likely to inherit.

genetics the study of heredity.

genital relating to the organs of reproduction.

genital herpes *see* herpes genitalis.

genital wart small, cauliflower-like swellings on the vulva or prepuce caused by a virus.

genitalia the organs of reproduction.

genitourinary relating to the function of the urinary and genital organs.

genome map pictorial representation showing the location of the genes on each chromosome.

genomics interdisciplinary field of science that is concerned with the structure, function, evolution and mapping of genomes.

genotype mapping of the individual genetic make-up.

genu the knee.

genupectoral position resting upon the knees and chest, with head down and hips elevated (*see* Fig. 41).

genus a classification of plants or animals by family or species grouping.

germ a common term applied to any microorganism. A substance, protoplasm, seed or spore capable of development into a new individual or whole organism.

German measles *see* rubella.

germicide an agent that kills germs.

gestation process of being carried or carrying in the womb; pregnancy.

gestational age the duration of pregnancy in completed weeks. It is calculated using the date of the first day of a woman's last menstrual period or by an ultrasound in the first trimester.

gestational diabetes mellitus (GDM) The World Health Organization defines GDM as hyperglycaemia first detected at any time during pregnancy; can be classified as either gestational diabetes mellitus or diabetes mellitus in pregnancy.

gestational hypertension (GH) the International Society for the Study of Hypertension in Pregnancy defines GH as average SBP ≥ 140 mmHg and/ or DBP ≥ 90 mmHg (phase 5) (after overnight rest in hospital, or after completion of a day assessment visit), developing after 20 weeks' gestation, without any evidence of multisystem dysfunction, e.g. kidneys, brain, liver, clotting.

gigantism abnormally large stature.

gingivitis inflammation of the mucous membranes and underlying soft tissues of the gum.

girdle a structure or band which encircles the body. The *pelvic girdle* is the bony encircling structure formed by the two innominate bones and the sacrum.

glabella the bony prominence formed by the joining of the frontal bones and supraorbital ridges.

gland a collection of tissue or specialised cells capable of secreting and excreting materials used to influence other bodily functions.

glans of clitoris erectile tissue at the end of the clitoris.

glans penis the expanded tip of the penis.

globin one of a class of proteins obtained from haemoglobin.

globulin a large group of plasma proteins (alpha, beta and gamma) that are characterised by their solubility in dilute salt solutions.

glomerulus a small rounded mass; the microscopic loops of capillaries, millions of which make up the kidney.

glossitis inflammation of the tongue.

glucagon hormones produced in the islets of Langerhans that stimulate conversion of glycogen to glucose.

glucocorticoid natural steroids that regulate carbohydrate, lipid and protein metabolism and inhibit the release of corticotropin. They are produced by the adrenal cortex.

glucose crystalline monosaccharide, dextrose, obtained by the incomplete hydrolysis of carbohydrates.

glucose-6-phosphate dehydrogenase (G6PD) an enzyme found in erythrocytes and other cells; a deficiency of this enzyme may trigger spontaneous haemolysis and ensuing jaundice.

glucose challenge test (GCT) a screening test used in pregnancy in which the body's response to a glucose load is compared to that of known healthy people. There should be an initial rise but a return to normal levels in 1 hour. Persistent elevation may be associated with diabetes.

glucose tolerance test (GTT) a diagnostic test for diabetes. Typically offered in pregnancy at 26–28 weeks' gestation or earlier if the woman has risk factors for diabetes in pregnancy.

glucosuria presence of glucose in the urine.

glucuronyl transferase a liver enzyme that hydrolyses fat-soluble bilirubin to an easily excreted water-soluble form.

gluteal pertaining to the buttocks or region of the buttocks.

gluteal muscle the largest muscle group in the buttocks.

glycerin a sweet, colourless fluid obtained from hydrolysed fats; used to carry medicine, moisten skin and lips and soften stools.

glycogen energy source formed from carbohydrates which are stored in the liver and muscles and converted into glucose when needed.

glycogenesis the formation of glycogen.

glycogenolysis the process of breaking down and liberation of glucagon from the liver to other tissues.

glycated haemoglobin a form of haemoglobin that can be measured to identify the 3-month average plasma glucose concentration. It is known as haemoglobin A1c, HbA1c, A1C or Hb1c.

glycosuria presence of sugar in the urine.

gnath-, gnatho- combining form denoting the jaw.

goitre swelling of the front of the neck caused by enlargement of the thyroid gland.

gonadotrophic hormone a hormone which stimulates activity in the gonads.

gonads a general term for glands or organs producing gametes; the testicles and ovaries.

gonococcus (PLURAL gonococci) the organism causing gonorrhoea, *Neisseria gonorrhoeae*.

gonorrhoea an easily treated sexually transmitted disease. If untreated, contact with the discharge during vaginal birth may cause ophthalmia neonatorum and blindness in the neonate.

Goodell's sign softening of the cervix uteri as a sign of pregnancy.

Graafian follicle the cystic structure surrounding the mature ovum on the surface

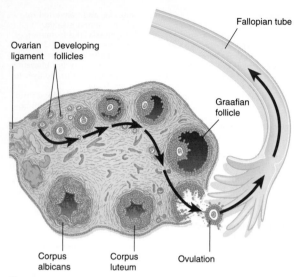

Figure 42
Graafian follicle

of the ovary which secretes oestrogen (*see* Fig. 42).

gram unit of weight of the metric system. Abbreviation 'g'.

gram staining a laboratory technique used to classify bacteria; having been exposed to alcohol, they either take up a staining lotion (*gram-positive*) or do not (*gram-negative*).

grand mal a form of epilepsy characterised by tonic–clonic seizures. The tonic phase is where the person's body becomes rigid, and the clonic phase is where there is jerking that the person cannot control themselves.

grand multipara a pregnant woman who has had four or more births. In some countries, five or more births is considered to be grand multiparity.

granulation an upward migration of newly formed capillaries and fibroblasts seen in wound healing.

granulosa cells epithelial cells lining the Graafian follicle.

grasp reflex the primitive reflex which can be triggered in the neonate by stroking the palm of the hands or sole of the foot. The fingers will curl around the stimulator and the resultant grasp is so strong as to enable the infant to be lifted.

gravid pregnant.

gravida a pregnant woman.

gravidarum gingivitis inflammation of the mucous membrane and underlying tissues of the gum; associated with pregnancy hormones.

grey syndrome a rare but serious side effect that occurs in newborn infants (especially those who are premature) following the intravenous administration of the antibiotic chloramphenicol. The condition occurs due to a lack of fully functional liver enzymes to metabolise the drug. Symptoms include vomiting, ashen grey colour of the skin and limp body tone.

grief physical manifestation of bereavement, separation or loss of a person or object with whom there is an emotional attachment.

groin the region between the abdomen and thighs.

gross large enough to be seen without magnification.

group antenatal care most of the antenatal care is provided in small groups of women, often of the same gestation but not always, rather than individual one-to-one care.

Group B streptococcal bacteria a common bacterium found in the gastrointestinal tract, vagina and urethra. Can be passed from mother to baby during labour and lead to infection (see early- and late-onset GBS).

group practice an establishment where several practitioners work together.

growth hormone a hormone directly influencing carbohydrate, fat and protein metabolism and promoting growth.

growth restriction failure of expected progress in growth in a fetus or neonate.

grunting abnormal respiratory sound noted on expiration indicating that the glottis has closed to the flow of air out of the lung, usually to prevent collapse of the lung. Heard in preterm infants suffering from respiratory distress syndrome.

gumma a lesion of tertiary syphilis.

gut the intestine; the embryonic digestive tract consists of foregut, midgut and hindgut.

Guthrie test the colloquial or generic name for the screening test to diagnose certain congenital conditions, e.g. phenylketonuria (see newborn screening test).

gyn-, gynae-, gyno- combining terms meaning woman.

gynaecoid woman-like; having female characteristics.

gynaecoid pelvis pelvis, the size and shape of which is ideal for childbirth.

gynaecology a branch of medicine devoted to the care of women, especially those with conditions of the reproductive organs and genitalia.

gynandromorphism the chromosomes of both genders are present in different tissues of the body, producing both male and female characteristics.

Hh

H symbol for hydrogen.

haem-, haemo- combining form denoting blood.

haemangioma a non-cancerous tumour composed of a mass of blood vessels.

haematemesis vomiting of blood.

haematocele collection of blood in a cavity.

haematocrit the percentage of whole blood occupied by red cells.

haematology the scientific study of the nature of blood, its function and diseases.

haematoma a mass formed by a collection of blood.

haematometra a collection of blood or menstrual fluid in the uterus.

haematosalpinx a collection of blood in the fallopian tube.

haematuria presence of blood in the urine.

haemoconcentration reduction of the fluid volume in the bloodstream.

haemodialysis a process in which blood is drained from the body a little at a time, mechanically filtered to remove impurities and returned.

haemodilution increase in the ratio of plasma to cells in the bloodstream. Normal physiology of early pregnancy is accompanied by a lowering of the haemoglobin.

haemoglobin the respiratory property of erythrocytes, consisting of four haem iron molecules linked to the protein globin and carrying out the dual functions of absorbing and releasing oxygen.

haemoglobin F (HbF) normal haemoglobin of the fetus, more fragile than adult haemoglobin and capable of absorbing oxygen at a lower tension.

haemoglobinopathy abnormal structure of one of the globin chains of the haemoglobin molecule that is genetic. Common haemoglobinopathies include sickle cell disease and thalassaemia.

haemolysin a substance which frees haemoglobin from red cells.

haemolysis the destruction of red cells and liberation of haemoglobin.

haemolytic having the ability to cause haemolysis.

haemolytic jaundice jaundice resulting from the destruction of excessive haemoglobin not required in extrauterine life. The resulting bile pigments remain in the circulation causing a yellow discolouration to the skin, until they can be removed by the maturing liver.

haemophilia a sex-linked recessive inherited disease of delayed clotting, carried by females but manifesting in males.

haemophilia B a hereditary haemophilial disease resulting from deficiency of pro-coagulant factor IX. Also called Christmas disease.

haemophilus a genus of bacteria dependent on blood pigments for growth.

haemopoiesis (SYNONYM haematopoiesis) the process of formation of blood.

haemoptysis coughing up of blood.

haemorrhage excessive loss of blood through injury or tissue damage.

haemorrhagic diathesis an abnormal bleeding tendency as in haemophilia, vitamin K deficiency or disseminated intravascular coagulation (DIC).

haemorrhagic disease of the newborn bleeding tendency in the newborn. Linked to deficiency of vitamin K in the neonate.

haemorrhoids (SYNONYM piles) the occurrence of varicose veins in the lower rectum and anus.

haemostasis the arrest of bleeding or haemorrhage.

haemostatic a drug or agent that arrests bleeding or haemorrhage.

hallucination sensory stimulus (visual, aural, tactile, etc.) perceived by an individual but unconnected to events outside the body.

hand presentation when the fetal hand lies lowest in the uterus in labour. This may occur when there is an uncorrected oblique lie allowing the arm and hand to prolapse into the vagina or as a compound presentation with the head.

haploid a cell nucleus containing half of the number of chromosomes.

hard chancre a 'crusty' ulcerated lesion at the site of the primary syphilitic infection.

hard palate the anterior part of the roof of the mouth located behind the teeth.

hare lip old, colloquial term for cleft or clefts in the upper lip.

harlequin ichthyosa a multicoloured congenital skin condition. The infant's skin is covered in scaly patches with red fissures between them which crack, allowing seepage of serous fluid.

Hartmann's solution a fluid administered intravenously to expand the volume of the circulating plasma.

Hb abbreviation for haemoglobin.

Hb electrophoresis (Hb EPG) part of the screening and diagnostic tests for thalassemia.

hCG *see* human chorionic gonadotrophin.

head box a perspex box with a cutout section to fit around the infant's neck. It is put over the head of a sick baby to deliver higher concentrations of oxygen than are available in the atmosphere.

health the World Health Organization (WHO) defines health as a 'state of complete physical, mental and social wellbeing and not merely the absence of disease or infirmity'. In more recent years, this statement has been modified to include the ability to lead a 'socially and economically productive life'.

health education method employed to enable individuals or collective populations to adopt strategies aimed at improvement in health through change and prevention of disease.

health literacy the degree to which people can obtain, process and understand basic information and services and make appropriate health decisions for themselves or their family.

Health Practitioners Disciplinary Tribunal hears and determines disciplinary proceedings brought against health practitioners.

health professional a person who has received training in healthcare.

heart the organ of circulation. A hollow muscular organ which functions as a pump maintaining circulation of the blood.

heartburn a burning sensation under the sternum caused by gastro-oesophageal reflux.

heart rate the speed at which the heart pumps blood around the body—normally 70–90 bpm in the adult and 110–160 bpm in an unborn baby.

Hegar's dilators a set of surgical instruments of increasing size used to dilate the cervix from the outside inwards.

Hegar's sign a possible sign of early pregnancy—on bimanual palpation the softening of the uterus allows the fingers to nearly meet above the level of the cervix.

hemicephalus condition where a fetus has only the lower half of its brain tissue present.

hemiplegia paralysis of one side of the body.

heparin a naturally occurring protein which prevents intravascular clotting.

hepatic pertaining to or involving the liver.

hepatitis inflammation of the liver. Can be caused by microorganisms, drugs, poisons or blood transfusions.

hepatitis B infectious disease caused by the hepatitis B virus (HBV) that affects the liver. It can cause both acute and chronic infections and can be transmitted from mother to baby. There are effective vaccines for hepatitis B.

hepatitis C infectious disease caused by the hepatitis C virus (HCV) that primarily affects the liver. It can be transmitted from mother to baby. There are currently no effective vaccines for hepatitis

C; treatments to clear the virus are now available, although they have not been tested during pregnancy.

hepatomegaly enlargement of the liver.

herbalist a therapist specialising in the medicinal properties of plants and who prescribes herbal infusions, tinctures, lotions and other preparations for medicinal use.

heredity the process by which traits, characteristics and diseases are passed from one generation to the next through the chromosomes.

hermaphrodite an individual of indeterminable gender, possessing both male and female genital organs. Usually not a preferred term for people with this condition; the preferred term is *intersex*.

hernia the abnormal protrusion of an organ beyond or outside of its normal containing walls due to a weakness in the containing wall.

heroin a white, crystalline powder, an acetyl derivative of morphine. It is a very powerful, habit-forming narcotic.

herpes an acute and highly contagious viral infection characterised by vesicle formation.

herpes genitalis (SYNONYM genital herpes) an infectious viral infection causing painful oozing vesicular lesions on the mucous membranes of the vulva or penis.

herpes gestationis a generalised itching and vesicular rash occurring during the second and third trimester of pregnancy.

herpes zoster (SYNONYM shingles) a painful condition caused by a virus where the eruption of lesions follows the course of a cutaneous nerve.

heterogenous different in kind or dissimilar.

heterotopic pregnancy (*see* ectopic pregnancy) a pregnancy occurring in an abnormal location, such as outside the uterine tubes or uterus.

heterozygous possessing dissimilar genes, e.g. a man whose blood group expression is rhesus positive, but who carries both positive and negative genes, and who is therefore able to father children that are either Rh-negative or Rh-positive.

Hg symbol for mercury, a liquid metal used in clinical thermometers and sphygmomanometers.

hiatus an abnormal space or opening.

hiatus hernia a small protrusion of the stomach into the oesophageal hiatus.

high forceps forceps that are applied when the fetal head is high—more than 2 cm above the ischial spines. Uncommonly used in contemporary practice.

hind waters the amniotic fluid behind and trapped by the fetal head.

Hirschsprung's disease congenital abnormality caused by absence of ganglion cells in a section of the colon or rectum; characterised by spasm in the ganglionic region and distension proximal to the defect. It may result in constipation, acute abdominal distension and obstruction.

hirsute excessive body hair.

histamine a protein liberated when tissue is injured or comes into contact with a foreign agent. It triggers arterial spasm, erythema, capillary dilation with increased permeability and oedema.

histology a branch of biology dealing with the microscopic structure of tissues and cells of organs.

history taking obtaining a detailed account of the woman's family history and past and present medical, surgical, obstetric, social and emotional health on which to base future care.

HIV *see* human immunodeficiency virus.

holistic taking into account the whole, all aspects of the person/situation.

holoacardius acephalus the abnormally formed twin of a normal fetus.

Homans' sign pain experienced in the calf and popliteal area on dorsiflexion of the foot. It is a positive sign of deep vein thrombosis.

homebirth labour and birth in the home; may be planned or unplanned.

homeopathy system of therapy in which treatment is by the administration of minute amounts of a substance that would usually cause the symptoms being treated.

homeostasis the tendency to remain in a state of equilibrium or balance; the status quo; remaining stable, as it was

homeothermic the ability of the body to maintain a stable temperature despite environmental conditions. This is not present in the neonate in the same way as an adult, which is why babies need to be kept warm.

homogeneous having the same qualities or being the same.

homologous chromosomes any two chromosomes that are identical in size and shape and carrying similar coding information in compatible sequence. Humans have 22 pairs and one different pair which denotes the gender of the individual.

homosexual 1. pertaining to the same sex or gender. 2. a person who is attracted to people of the same sex.

homosexuality sexual attraction between people of the same sex.

homozygous having two genes which carry the same characteristic, e.g. a man who is homozygous Rh-positive carries two Rh-positive genes which means that he will always pass an Rh-positive gene on to any children he has.

hormones chemicals produced by endocrine glands and secreted into the bloodstream. They act to bring about specific regulatory effects on body parts remote from their origin.

hourglass constriction 1. an encircling contraction of an organ causing it to be divided more or less into two compartments. 2. contraction of the uterus occurring in the third stage of labour causing entrapment of the placenta; may be a cause of postpartum haemorrhage.

hourglass uterus an abnormal stricture occurring at the junction of the upper and lower uterine segment in which a band of circular muscles in the uterus contract independently causing lack of progress in labour.

Huhner test fertility test carried out on seminal fluid withdrawn from the vaginal fornix 1 hour after intercourse. It is examined for sperm activity and survival.

human chorionic gonadotrophin (hCG) a hormone produced by the trophoblast after conception. Its action is to maintain the corpus luteum and prevent menstruation thereby ensuring the survival of the pregnancy.

human immunodeficiency virus (HIV) a slow-acting retrovirus contained in blood and body fluids which impacts on the immune system of the body. Main routes of transmission are sexual intercourse, blood transfusion, organ transplantation, vertically from mother to infant in utero/at birth or through breastfeeding.

human placental lactogen (HPL) a growth-type hormone secreted by the placenta affecting carbohydrate metabolism.

human papillomavirus (HPV) common sexually transmitted infection which usually causes no symptoms and goes away by itself, but can sometimes cause cancer in the long term. HPV is responsible for almost all cases of genital warts and cervical cancer and contributory to a number of other concerns (vaginal, anal, penile).

humerus the bone of the upper arm.

Hutchinson's triad a term describing three linked indicators of congenital syphilis. The baby is born with interstitial keratitis and deafness, and will develop notched teeth.

hyaline a clear vitreous protein material found in various body tissues including the lungs.

hyaline membrane disease see respiratory distress syndrome (RDS).

hydatidiform mole degeneration of the placenta and proliferation of the

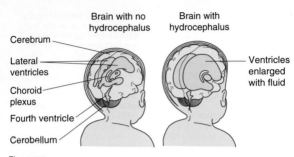

Figure 43
Hydrocephalus
Illustration by Alan Laver

trophoblast into hydropic vesicles resembling a bunch of grapes.

hydra-, hydro- combining form denoting water or hydrogen.

hydraemia a disproportionate increase in the volume of plasma to red cells in the blood.

hydralazine an antihypertensive drug used in the management of severe hypertension.

hydramnios normal volume of amniotic fluid.

hydration absorption of water.

hydrocele accumulation of fluid in the sac or tunica vaginalis of the testes. A common non-pathological condition in the neonate, which resolves spontaneously.

hydrocephalus enlargement of the head with water. A congenital defect caused by accumulation of cerebrospinal fluid, leading to distension of

the ventricles and damage to the brain tissue (*see* Fig. 43).

hydrochloric acid a naturally occurring chemical component of gastric juices and essential to the digestion of food. Aspiration of hydrochloric acid into the lung causes Mendelson's syndrome.

hydrocortisone an adrenocortical steroid.

hydrogen the lightest of the known gases which combines with oxygen to form water, H_2O.

hydrogen ions the positively electric charged nucleus. The pH of the blood is determined by the concentration of hydrogen ions.

hydronephrosis retention of urine with back pressure, dilation of the renal pelvis and destruction of the kidney substance secondary to obstruction.

hydrops fetalis severe and generalised oedema, jaundice and anaemia of the fetus due to Rh incompatibility; may result in fetal death.

hydrops gravidarum oedema occurring in pregnancy.

hydrosalpinx fluid distension of the fallopian tubes.

hygiene a group of practical approaches to attaining and maintaining health by preventing the multiplication of microorganisms.

hygroma a cystic lymph-filled cavity occurring as a congenital malformation.

hymen a membranous structure partially blocking the orifice of the vagina before sexual intercourse.

hyoscine (scopolamine) drug used to depress the central nervous system which reduces salivary secretions and has amnesic properties.

hyper- combining term denoting excess or above normal.

hyperbilirubinaemia high blood levels of bilirubin, often seen in the neonate due to rapid haemolysis of fetal haemoglobin. Very high levels can cause kernicterus and brain damage.

hypercalcaemia excess of calcium in the circulation.

hypercapnia excess of carbon dioxide in the circulation.

hyperdactyly a developmental anomaly characterised by the presence of more than the usual number of fingers or toes.

hyperemesis excessive vomiting.

hyperemesis gravidarum excessive vomiting in pregnancy. This can be a serious problem resulting in electrolyte imbalance.

hyperglycaemia excess of glucose in the circulation.

hyperglycaemia in pregnancy high levels of glucose in pregnancy which indicates a number of specific conditions including: impaired fasting glucose and impaired glucose tolerance (pre-diabetes), preexisting type 1 diabetes, preexisting type 2 diabetes (either previously diagnosed or diagnosed during pregnancy) and gestational diabetes (developing during pregnancy).

hyperkalaemia excess of potassium in the circulation.

hyperlactation secretion of milk from the breasts beyond the normal duration of breastfeeding.

hypernatraemia excess of sodium in the circulation.

hyperphenylalaninaemia a positive indicator of the condition phenylketonuria in which there are high levels of the protein phenylalanine in the blood. If untreated it can lead to brain damage.

hyperplasia growth by increase in cell numbers.

hyperpyrexia a body temperature over 40°C.

hypersensitivity excess immunological response to a drug or allergen not experienced by the majority of people.

hypertension abnormally high blood pressure.

hypertension in pregnancy the International Society for the Study of Hypertension in Pregnancy defines hypertension in pregnancy as a systolic blood pressure equal to or greater than 140 mmHg and/or diastolic blood pressure (Korotkoff V) equal to or greater than 90 mmHg. It is noted that these blood pressures should be confirmed by repeated readings using mercury sphygmomanometry over several hours in a clinic or day assessment unit or after a rest in hospital.

hyperthyroidism excessive secretion of thyroid hormones into the blood resulting in raised metabolic rate, hyperactivity, tachycardia, sweating, emaciation, tremor and exophthalmos.

hypertonia increase to excess in the tone or tension of muscles or blood vessels.

hypertonic solution a solution with an osmotic pressure greater than physiologic saline.

hypertrophy increase in the size of an organ by a process of enlargement of its cells.

hyperventilation abnormally rapid breathing with excessive removal of carbon dioxide; hypocapnia.

hypnosis a state of altered consciousness. The person acts under the influence of a taught suggestion. Can be used as a method for coping with labour.

hypnotherapy treatment based on hypnosis. Some women can manage pain in labour by altering their level of consciousness.

hypnotic a drug which induces sleep.

hypo- combining term meaning below normal or under.

hypocalcaemia reduction in the amount of calcium in the circulation.

hypocapnia diminished carbon dioxide in the blood.

hypochlorhydria reduction in the amount of hyperchloric acid in the gastric juice.

hypochondrium the right or left upper lateral region of the abdomen, beneath the ribs.

hypochromic reduction in colour or pigment. Description of the iron-deficient erythrocyte as seen in anaemia.

hypodermic 1. subcutaneous. 2. a substance or medicine injected or introduced beneath the skin.

hypofibrinogenaemia a reduction in the plasma level of fibrinogen.

hypogastric relating to the hypogastrium or pubic region.

hypogastric artery a branch from the internal iliac artery which in fetal life carries deoxygenated blood and communicates directly with the umbilical artery.

hypoglycaemia a reduction of glucose in the circulation.

hypognathia having an abnormally small lower jaw.

hypomagnesaemia abnormally low magnesium content of the blood, manifested chiefly by neuromuscular hyperirritability.

hypopituitarism clinical condition resulting in reduced secretion from the anterior pituitary gland. It may occur secondary to severe postpartum haemorrhage when there is pituitary necrosis (*see* Sheehan's syndrome), with atrophy of the gonads, thyroid and adrenal glands and secondary infertility.

hypoplasia arrested development of a tissue or organ.

hypospadias a congenital malformation in which the urethra opens on the side surface of the penis or into the vaginal canal.

hypostasis formation of deposits or sedimentation.

hypostatic 1. resulting from hypostasis. 2. a state of being suppressed. In genetics this relates to the genetic characteristic or function that is overshadowed by another gene (of the matched pair), affecting or influencing its functional ability.

hypostatic pneumonia pneumonia developing in the sick patient whose respirations are shallow and who is immobile for long periods.

hypotension abnormally low vessel tension resulting in reduction of blood pressure.

hypothalamus the region of the brain forming the floor of the third ventricle. It controls sympathetic and parasympathetic nervous systems, pituitary activity and various other bodily functions.

hypothermia subnormal body temperature.

hypothermia neonatorum body temperature below 35°C usually as a result of the infant being born in a cool room or inadequately cared for or dried at birth.

hypothesis a conjecture or theory put forward to account for known facts or as a basis for discussion.

hypothyroidism reduction in the functional state of the thyroid gland and insufficiency in production of hormones resulting in cretinism in a child or myxoedema in an adult.

hypotonia reduction in muscle tone.

hypotonic solution a solution that is weaker than physiologic saline and contains less than 0.9 g of sodium chloride per 100 mL.

hypoventilation reduction in respiratory effort.

hypovolaemia marked reduction in the circulating blood volume.

hypovolaemic shock shock or collapsed state caused by excessive loss of blood or plasma.

hypoxia reduction in oxygen level required for normal physiological function.

hypoxic-ischemic encephalopathy (HIE) a serious birth complication which is caused by oxygen deprivation to the brain.

hysterectomy surgical removal of the uterus.

hysteria a term formerly used widely in psychiatry. It is not a term used in contemporary clinical practice.

hystero-oophorectomy excision of the uterus and one or both ovaries.

hystero-salpingectomy excision of the uterus and the uterine tubes after instillation of a contrast medium.

hysterosalpingogram a way to assess the patency of the fallopian tubes using the injection of a dye through the cervix and into the uterus and visualisation by X-ray.

hystero-salpingo contrast sonography (HyCoSy) a way to assess the patency of the fallopian tubes using the injection of a dye through the cervix and into the uterus and visualisation by ultrasound.

hysterotomy surgical incision into the uterus made for termination of a pregnancy after 12 weeks' but before 20 weeks' gestation.

hysteroscopy a procedure where a small camera is passed through the cervix into the lower end of the uterus to view the lining of the woman's uterus. The cervix needs to be dilated for the camera to pass into the uterus. The procedure is carried out under anaesthetic.

iatrogenic a pathological condition caused by treatment given for another condition.

ichthyosis increased or aberrant keratinisation of the skin which results in non-inflammatory scaling.

icterus neonatorum jaundice (yellow skin membranes and sclera) of the newborn.

idiopathic primary; of unknown cause.

idiosyncrasy a peculiarity of character or temperament which makes an individual different from others.

Ig symbol for particular gamma globulins (Ig A, D, E, G and M) which offer immunological protection against specific organisms.

ileocaecal valve the valve situated at the junction of the ileum with the caecum that partially prevents reflux.

ileum the terminal section of the small intestine.

ileus intestinal obstruction caused by paralysis of the ileum in which peristalsis is arrested and distension occurs.

iliac pertaining to the ilium or ilial region.

iliac crest the thickened expanded upper border of the hip bone.

iliac fossa the wide shallow depression on the inner surface of the ilium.

iliococcygeal referring to the ilium and coccyx.

iliopectineal referring to the ilium and pubic bone.

ilium the superior widened portion of the hip bone.

immature not yet fully developed.

immature baby a baby born prematurely, before body systems are developed enough to ensure its survival outside the uterus.

immersion putting into or covering with water. Women may use a bath or birth pool in labour to reduce pain and enhance coping mechanisms by equalising internal uterine and external pressure.

immobilisation removal of capacity of movement.

immune protected against a particular disease.

immune response a reaction involving a specific antibody response to an antigen.

immune system the body's natural defence against disease, comprising the biochemical complex of antibodies and T-cells, etc., which respond to and protect the body from some infections.

immunisation the active process of developing immunity; the giving of substances in the hope of helping a person develop immunity to one or more diseases.

immunity the ability of an organism to mount an antibody response to resist disease.

immunodeficient the failure of the immune system to protect the body from damage by common pathogenic organisms.

immunoglobulin (Ig) proteins or gamma globulins having known antibody activity (IgA, IgD, IgE, IgG, IgM).

immunologic pregnancy test a means of detecting the presence of a pregnancy by measuring the increased concentration of human chorionic gonadotrophin in urine.

immunoprophylaxis a process of hastening immunity by giving live weakened

pathogens to an individual or passive immunity through transfer of antibodies made in another body.

impaction being lodged or wedged into a confined space.

impaired glucose tolerance (IGT) abnormally raised fasting blood glucose levels or failure to return to normal parameters within 2 hours of a glucose tolerance test (GTT). May be due to gestational diabetes.

imperforate without the normal opening.

imperforate anus congenital occlusion of the anal opening (*see* Fig. 44).

imperforate hymen the absence of a natural opening in the hymen membrane covering the vagina. The barrier prevents escape of menstrual blood.

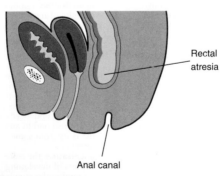

Rectal atresia

Anal canal

Figure 44
Imperforate anus

impetigo streptococcal or staphylococcal infection of the skin characterised by vesicles which burst exposing erythematous areas. Severe affliction is known as pemphigus neonatorum and is a highly infectious condition.

impetigo herpetiformis a skin condition starting in pregnancy. It resembles a pustular psoriasis with lesions in the genitofemoral area which may spread to other areas.

implant 1. to embed or introduce into the body tissue. 2. something which is embedded or introduced into the body tissue.

implantation 1. the act of implanting, as in the embedding of the fertilised ovum into the endometrium. 2. the enclosing of drugs such as hormones or radioactive substances in rods, which are then buried under the skin enabling slow release for treatment of certain conditions.

impotent incapable of performing the sexual act.

impregnate to make pregnant.

intracytoplasmic sperm injection (ICSI) fertility technique where a single sperm is selected and directly injected into an egg.

in utero within the uterus.

intrauterine insemination (IUI) a procedure that involves semen being inserted through the cervix into the uterus close to the time of ovulation to achieve conception.

in vitro literally, in glass. Used in reference to a process of culture or growth within a test tube.

in vitro fertilisation (IVF) fertilisation of the ovum outside the woman's body. Sperm and ovum are removed from their donors, mixed in a glass dish and after fertilisation has occurred the conceptus is reintroduced into the uterus for implantation and development to occur.

inborn characteristics that are inherited or congenital.

inborn error of metabolism an inherited genetic characteristic whereby the infant is unable to synthesise foods into simple compounds for ingestion and energy production due to lack of specific enzymes, as in, for example, phenylketonuria and galactosaemia.

inbreeding mating between closely related family members permitting genes and traits to be expressed most strongly in the offspring.

incarcerate enclose, confine or imprison.

incarceration of the retroverted gravid uterus pregnancy conceived with the uterus in the retroverted position which has failed to spontaneously correct, leading to entrapment of the enlarging uterus in the hollow of the sacrum by the sacral promontory.

incest sexual intercourse which is illegal because it is between close members of a family who by law are unable to marry.

incision a cutting into.

incompatibility antagonistic chemical changes resulting when two substances are put together that are not conducive to successful combination.

incompetence inadequacy at the level of normal functional performance.

incomplete miscarriage describes the situation where some products of conception remain in the uterus after some have been expelled. Surgical removal may be offered to prevent the possibility of infection.

incontinence involuntary and inappropriate passage of urine or faeces due to inability to control the urethral or anal sphincter muscles.

incoordinate lacking the harmonious working relationship of various parts.

incubate to artificially heat as a means of bringing about development.

incubation the process of development.

incubation period the time from exposure to an infectious disease to exhibition of symptoms.

incubator 1. a cabinet with controlled temperature used for assisting growth of bacteria or hatching of eggs. 2. a chamber that is closely regulated for temperature, humidity and oxygen in which sick or low birth weight babies are cared for.

independent midwife (SYNONYM privately practising midwife) a midwife who is self-employed and offers midwifery care to women.

indigenous occurring naturally in a certain locality.

indirect Coombs' test a screening test performed to detect free antibodies in blood. An Rh-negative mother may have this test done (or the direct Coombs' test done on cord blood) to detect antibodies indicating that the neonate is Rh-positive.

induced abortion intentional termination of pregnancy by drugs or surgical means.

induction the act of bringing about a particular action. Applied to procedures such as abortion, anaesthesia or labour.

induction of labour intentional stimulation of a pregnant uterus to initiate labour using drugs, mechanical or surgical means.

inertia an ineffective level of activity or sluggishness.

inevitable abortion having reached a stage at which prevention of an abortion is unavoidable.

infant a child up to 12 months of age.

infant death death of a child within the first year of life.

infant mortality rate the number of deaths per year in children under the age of 1 year per 1000 live births.

infanticide the murder of an infant.

infantile 1. pertaining to the period of infancy. 2. having characteristics like those exhibited in infancy.

infantile paralysis historical term for *poliomyelitis*.

infarct ischaemia or necrosis of tissue due to inadequate blood supply.

infarction the development of an infarct.

infected septic miscarriage termination of pregnancy complicated by invasion of the genital tract with pathogenic organisms. This can be life-threatening; antibiotics and evacuation of the uterus are required. Also known as *septic abortion*.

infection the pathogenic state caused by entry of a microorganism into a host.

infectious disease a contagious illness caused by an organism invading a host.

infective mastitis bacterial infection of the breast because a blocked milk duct causes milk to pool in the breast. This forms an ideal environment for bacteria growth and can lead to an infection.

inferior below or under.

inferior longitudinal sinus a blood vessel passing around and below the sagittal suture between the parietal bones of the skull.

inferior vena cava the large blood vessel at the lower edge of the falx cerebri.

infertility an involuntary inability to conceive.

infibulation the practice of surgical closure of the labia majora by sewing them together to partially seal the vagina, leaving only a small hole for the passage of urine and menstrual blood. It is usually performed at the same time as female genital mutilation (FGM; removal of the clitoris). The labia minora are often also removed.

infiltrate entry and dispersal of agents into tissue.

inflammation reaction of tissues to injury. Characteristic responses are heat, swelling, redness, pain and loss or reduction of functional ability.

influenza an acute respiratory infection caused by a virus.

informed consent permission for treatment voluntarily obtained from women; the woman must have received a detailed explanation of what is involved, including risks and benefits, in a manner that she is able to understand.

informed refusal declining of a procedure or treatment which has been offered to a woman, after her consideration of the benefits, risks and alternatives.

infra- a prefix meaning below.

infundibulum (PLURAL infundibula) resembling a funnel; a funnel-shaped passage, e.g. the distal end of the fallopian tube.

infusion 1. extraction of the soluble properties of a

substance by means of soaking in water, but without boiling.
2. slow injection of solution into the body by the intravenous or subcutaneous route.

ingestion 1. the taking in of food or other substances by the oral route. 2. the process by which specialised cells take in or envelop bacteria.

inguinal (LATIN *inguen*) pertaining to the groin region.

inguinal canal a small channel running obliquely downwards through the abdominal wall and towards the groin which enables passage of nerves and ligaments. It is also the migratory route taken by the testes in their descent into the scrotal sac.

inguinal hernia descent or herniation of abdominal content into the inguinal canal.

inhalation the process of breathing in a gas or vapour for medicinal or therapeutic purposes.

inheritance characteristics genetically acquired from a parent.

inhibin a testicular hormone.

inhibition a restraining of action in an organ or cell.

iniencephaly a congenital anomaly where: the foramen magnum is enlarged; there is absence of the laminal and spinous processes of the cervical, dorsal and sometimes lumbar vertebrae; and the brain and much of the spinal cord occupy a single cavity. The vertebrae may be reduced in number and irregularly fused.

injection the introduction of fluids into the skin, muscle, blood vessel, spinal cord or any body cavity.

inlet the entrance to a cavity, e.g. the pelvic inlet or entrance to the true pelvis.

innate present at birth, hereditary, genetically determined.

inner cell mass the compact group of cells that are part of the blastocyst from which the fetus and amniotic membranes develop.

innervation the distribution or supply of nerves to a part.

innominate literally, nameless. The *innominate bone* is the collective name given to the bones of the pelvic girdle. It combines the fusion of the ilium, ischium and os pubis (*see* Fig. 45).

inoculate to introduce agents derived from a diseased animal or plant into the body of a healthy person for the purpose of giving protection against that same disease, e.g. a vaccine.

inquest a legal enquiry for the purpose of determining the cause of sudden, violent or unexplained death.

insemination 1. the planting of seed. 2. the introduction of seminal fluid into the female genital tract for the purpose of achieving conception.

insertion the anchorage point of a muscle or the attachment of an organ to its support.

insidious gradual development or progression of a condition

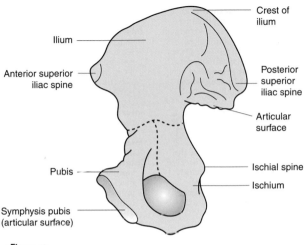

Figure 45
Innominate bone

or disease so as to be almost imperceptible.

insomnia inability to sleep.

inspection to look at or examine visually, e.g. before abdominal palpation.

inspiration inhalation, drawing in of breath.

instillation introduction of a liquid into a cavity or canal drop by drop.

instrument a tool with a specific purpose.

instrumental birth the use of an instrument to aid birth, e.g. ventouse, forceps.

insufficiency the inability to perform at the optimal level of function.

insufflation the introduction of gas, powder or vapour into a body cavity by blowing or positive pressure.

insulin 1. the hypoglycaemic hormone secreted by the beta cells of the islets of Langerhans in the pancreas which regulates carbohydrate and fat metabolism. 2. a synthetic drug which replaces endogenous insulin.

intelligence quotient (IQ) a numerical rating used to designate a person's cognitive skill (understanding) as compared to the average for age and social situation.

intermittent preventive treatment in pregnancy (IPTp) is a public health intervention aimed at treating and preventing malaria episodes in pregnant women.

intensive care unit a designated area where the critically ill can be observed and monitored constantly and receive additional supportive care and therapy from specially qualified persons.

intention to practise documentation completed by each midwife at the commencement of work and annually, ensuring the availability of a local and up-to-date list of midwives competent to practise. This terminology is used mostly in the United Kingdom.

inter- prefix denoting between.

intercellular between cells.

intercostal between the ribs.

intercourse communication or interaction. *Sexual intercourse* (coitus) is penetration of the vagina by the penis and ejaculation.

interface a surface that forms a boundary between two opposing units.

interferon a protein formed by cells in response to a virus which prevents future viral replication and can induce resistance to a range of other viruses.

interleukin-8 a low-molecular-weight protein involved in cell-to-cell communication, coordination of antibodies, T-cell immune interactions and the inflammatory process; it may have some effect on the commencement of labour.

intermenstrual referring to the time between menstrual periods.

intermittent occurring at intervals or periodically.

intermittent positive pressure ventilation (IPPV) mechanical ventilation of the lungs, often employed in babies with severe respiratory distress syndrome.

internal os the innermost opening or mouth at the junction of the uterine cavity with the cervix.

internal podalic version a procedure where the operator's hand is introduced into the uterus to apply pressure to convert a malpresentation that cannot be born easily (e.g. shoulder presentation) to one which may be more safely born vaginally (e.g. breech) by bringing the feet down so that they are the presenting part (*see* internal version).

internal rotation of the fetus in the second stage of labour, when the cervix is fully dilated, this is part of the mechanism performed by the fetus as it adapts to the changing shape and diameters of the birth canal.

internal version manipulation of the fetus in utero to alter the lie from oblique to longitudinal when the breech presents or to correct a brow presentation. One hand is inserted into the uterus while the other works externally over the abdomen.

International Confederation of Midwives (ICM) a global organisation of midwives associations with members in more than 120 countries.

interrupted not continuous. An *interrupted suture* is a type of wound closure in which each stitch is tied and cut before the next one is applied.

intersex a term referring to individuals who have characteristics (anatomical, chromosomal and/or hormonal) that differ from conventional or medical understanding of female and male bodies.

interspinous situated between or connecting bony protrusions.

interstitial relating to the space between organs filled by fine connective tissue.

interstitial fibroid a fibroid which develops and is located within the intercellular connective tissue layers of the uterus.

interstitial mastitis inflammation of the connective tissue between the ducts of the breast.

interstitial tubal pregnancy a pregnancy which has implanted in the narrowest part of the fallopian tube.

intertrigo an inflammation of the skin where two skin surfaces rub or press against each other trapping moisture, bacteria, yeast or fungus in the folds.

intervillous situated between villi.

intestinal flora the naturally occurring non-pathogenic microorganisms found in the large intestine and responsible for the manufacture of vitamin K and other useful substances.

intestinal obstruction spasmodic and inflammatory constriction of the gut causing blockage and preventing material from passing through. It causes pain, distension and tenderness and constitutes a medical emergency often requiring emergency surgery.

intestine the part of the digestive tract extending from the stomach to the anus.

intimate partner violence (IPV) the World Health Organization defines IPV as any behaviour within an intimate relationship that causes physical, psychological or sexual harm to those in the relationship; is now recognised as a global public health issue (*see also* domestic violence). It is also referred to as gender-based violence.

intra- prefix denoting within or inward.

intra-abdominal pressure pressure within the abdomen from accumulation of gases, faecal material, infection or pregnancy.

intracerebral haemorrhage bleeding inside the brain (*see* Fig. 46).

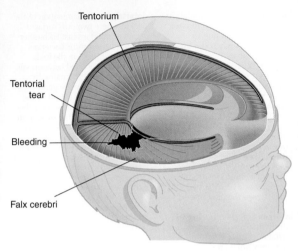

Figure 46
Intracerebral haemorrhage

intracranial inside the head.
intracranial haemorrhage
bleeding within the skull; can
occur in the neonate
following an instrumental or
vaginal breech birth.
intracranial pressure a rise
from the normal pressure
level caused by an
accumulation of blood or fluid
under the skull, recognised by
falling pulse rate and rising
blood pressure, increased
restlessness and a decrease in
the level of consciousness.
intradermal into or within the
skin. An *intradermal injection*
is one given between the

epidermis and the dermis (*see*
Fig. 47).
intramenstrual pain uterine
pain between menstrual
periods; there may be an
association with ovulation.
intramuscular into or within a
muscle. An *intramuscular
injection* is one given into a
muscle (*see* Fig. 48).
intrapartum occurring during
childbirth, that is, labour and
birth.
intrapartum fetal death fetal
death occurring during
labour.
intrapartum haemorrhage
bleeding from the genital

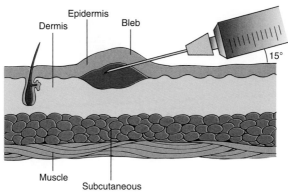

Figure 47
Intradermal injection technique

tract during labour; may be associated with placenta praevia or abruptio placentae.

intrauterine within the uterus.

intrauterine contraceptive device (IUCD) mechanical device inserted within the uterine cavity which prevents implantation or development of the fertilised embryo (*see* Fig. 49).

intrauterine death (IUD) death of the fetus while in the uterus.

intrauterine growth restriction (IUGR) (previously known as *intrauterine growth retardation*) where the fetus does not develop in accordance with recognised growth curves with regard to increasing weight, size and bone length.

intravascular within the blood vessels.

intravascular coagulation clotting of blood within the blood vessels. They may then cause other vessels to become obstructed (e.g. in the kidney) and damage in that organ may be permanent. The clotting factors will become unbalanced and haemorrhage is possible.

intravenous (IV, iv) within or into a vein.

intravenous infusion (IVI) introduction of a fluid into the body (e.g. for hydration) to increase circulating volume before introduction of a potentially hypotensive drug, as a circulatory expander, or for nutritional purposes.

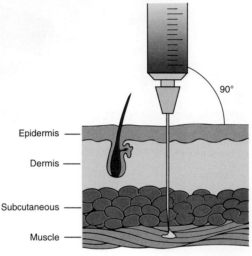

Figure 48
Intramuscular injection technique

intravenous injection a drug or medicine introduced directly into the circulatory system so that the time for it to take effect is short.

intraventricular haemorrhage bleeding into the ventricles deep within the brain. It can happen to preterm infants or those experiencing a traumatic birth.

intrinsic situated or produced within a part, relating to inherent factor within itself.

intrinsic factor a substance produced by the stomach which, when combined with properties of food (vitamin B_{12}, the extrinsic factor), is essential to prevent pernicious anaemia.

introitus an entrance; the term is often used to refer to the opening of the vagina.

intubation the introduction of a tube into a hollow organ. *Endotracheal intubation* is used to achieve mechanical ventilation in cases of neonatal asphyxia or in association with induction of anaesthesia.

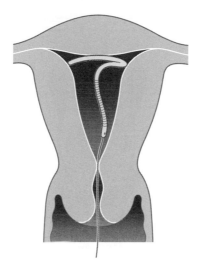

Figure 49
Intrauterine contraceptive device (IUCD)

---

intussusception the prolapse
of the bowel either into itself
or through the rectum.
invasion the process whereby a
disease or pathogen enters,
infects and damages the body.
inverse, inverted located in the
opposite position from that
which it is normally expected;
turned inwards or upside
down.
inversion turning inside out.
Uterine inversion is a rare but
serious complication of the
third stage of labour (*see*
Fig. 50); it causes profound

shock and may be fatal if not
corrected immediately.
inverted *see* inverse.
involuntary acting
independently of will or
conscious control.
involution a process of
regression which some organs
undergo, having fulfilled their
intended function.
involution of the uterus return
of the uterus to its
non-pregnant condition
(*see* Fig. 51).
ion an atom or group of atoms
which by application of an

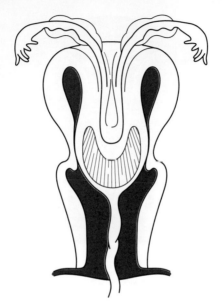

Figure 50
Inversion of the uterus

energy source can gain or lose electrons and be rendered capable of conducting electricity.

IPV *see* intimate partner violence.

iris the coloured portion of the eye. In the centre is the pupil which contracts and dilates to regulate the entrance of light into the eye.

iritis inflammation of the iris of the eye.

iron an organic metal used in the form of salts in medicines for the treatment of anaemia. It is essential in the manufacture of haemoglobin.

ischaemia diminution of blood supply to an area of the body.

ischaemic necrosis tissue death occurring secondary to lack of an adequate blood supply.

ischial relating to the ischium.

ischial spine the bony prominence on the ischium

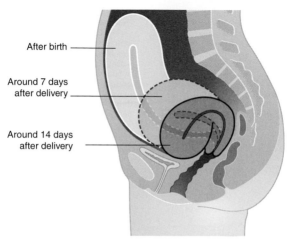

After birth

Around 7 days
after delivery

Around 14 days
after delivery

Figure 51
Involution of the uterus

which protrudes into the
pelvic cavity.
ischial tuberosity the rounded
lower border of the ischium
on which the body rests when
sitting.
ischiocavernosus muscle
muscle from the ischium to
the clitoris or penis.
ischiococcygeus muscle
muscle from the ischium to
the coccyx.
ischium the inferior and
posterior dense portion of the
innominate bone upon which
the body rests when in a
sitting position.

islets of Langerhans the
endocrine structures of the
pancreas which produce insulin.
Insulin controls carbohydrate
metabolism. In the disease
diabetes mellitus the islets fail.
isoimmunisation sensitisation of
a species with antigens from
the same species. This can
occur in mismatched blood
transfusion or where a woman
is Rh-negative and the fetus
Rh-positive. Fetal blood cells
can pass into the maternal
circulation which may cause
the woman to produce
antibodies against the foreign

cells. The antibodies she
produces can cross the placenta,
enter the fetal circulation and
cause haemolysis.

isolation separation of an
infective individual from the
remainder of the community
to contain and prevent the
spread of a communicable
disease to others.

isotonic relating to uniformity
of strength.

isotonic solution solution
containing the same osmotic
pressure as the tissue with
which it is compared and
capable of promoting or
maintaining its normal state
or function. Physiologic
normal saline is isotonic with
plasma.

isthmus the constricted part or
neck of an organ.

Jj

Jacquemier's sign blue discolouration of the vaginal lining seen in early pregnancy and taken as one of the presumptive signs.

jaundice yellow discolouration of the skin, mucous membranes and sclera due to hyperbilirubinaemia.

jejunum portion of the small intestine which extends from the duodenum to the ileum.

joint the point at which two or more bones meet.

joint instability the effects of the hormones progesterone and relaxin on the joints in pregnancy causing them to soften and have an increased range of movement, e.g. the sacroiliac joint and the symphysis pubis.

joule (J) the international unit of energy measurement in food.

jugular relating to the neck or region above the clavicle.

justice ethical principle which recognises fairness and equality of treatment for all.

justo minor abnormally small in all dimensions. A term applied to the perfectly formed but small gynaecoid pelvis.

juvenile young adult, youth.

juxta- prefix denoting nearness or proximity to, as in *juxtaposition*.

Kk

K symbol for potassium.

kallikrein a proteolytic enzyme present in several body fluids that releases kallidin.

kangaroo care a method of caring for the neonate derived from the Australian marsupial in which the immature offspring is carried and suckled in a pouch on the mother's abdomen. It has been found to be physiologically beneficial.

Kaposi's sarcoma multiple, idiopathic haemorrhagic sarcoma lesions, often seen as a feature of AIDS.

karyo- combining form denoting nucleus.

karyogenesis formation and development of cell nuclei.

karyotype the total characteristics including numbers, size and form of chromosomes and their grouping in a cell nucleus.

Kegel exercises specific exercises designed to strengthen the pelvic floor (pubococcygeus) muscles.

Kell blood group a family of antigens found in erythrocytes in a small percentage of the population (K, k, Kp^a, Kp^b and Ku).

keloid fibrous tissue hyperplasia formed at the site of a scar.

keratin an albuminous substance forming the base of all horny tissues (hair, nails, feathers, etc.).

kernicterus bilirubin hyper pigmentation of the basal ganglia of the brain with destruction of nerve cells, seen as a complication of severe neonatal jaundice caused by Rh isoimmunisation.

Kernig's sign pain and spasm of the hamstring muscles resulting in an inability of a supine patient to straighten the leg when it is flexed at the knee and hip—a sign of meningitis.

ketoacidosis accumulation of ketone bodies and acetic acid in the blood. This can occur when the body is starved of a ready supply of energy and breaks down body stores of fats leading to the production of toxic metabolites.

ketone body acetone formed by the metabolism of fats.

ketonuria the presence of ketone bodies in the urine.

ketosis condition in which excessive amounts of ketones are present in the body.

ketotic presence of ketones in the body as indicated by acidic expired air and ketonuria.

kick chart a graphical record made by a pregnant woman indicating the number of fetal movements counted during a

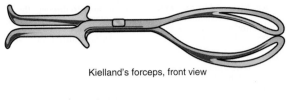

Kielland's forceps, front view

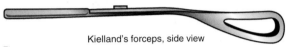

Kielland's forceps, side view

Figure 52
Kielland's forceps
Illustration by Alan Laver

designated time period; previously used as an assessment of fetal wellbeing but now mostly replaced by maternal fetal movement pattern awareness.

Kielland's forceps an obstetric forceps, characterised by reduced curvature of the blades and interlocking handles (*see* Fig. 52). Used for mid-cavity application and rotation of the fetal head.

killed vaccine an injection of dead microorganisms to which the body responds by producing antibodies.

kilo- prefix indicating 'one thousand'.

kinase an enzyme that catalyses transfer of phosphate from adenosine triphosphate to an acceptor.

kinin any of a group of polypeptides capable of initiating capillary wall activity. Bradykinin (causes relaxation of capillary walls) is mainly hypotensive while angiotensin (causes constriction of capillary walls) is hypertensive.

Kleihauer test a blood test performed on the Rh-negative woman to detect the presence of fetal cells in the maternal circulation. Where detected and the fetus is identified as Rh-positive, anti-D immunoglobulin is offered to the woman in an attempt to prevent isoimmunisation.

Klinefelter's syndrome a clinical syndrome in males characterised by having an additional sex chromosome (XXY instead of XY). The testes fail to mature at puberty and there may be female characteristics such as the development of breasts.

Klisic test used in the clinical examination of an infant to detect congenital hip dysplasia. The examiner places their middle finger on the greater trochanter and index finger on the anterior superior iliac spine. Usually, an imaginary line drawn between the two fingers will point to the umbilicus. In a dislocated hip the line points between the pubis and umbilicus.

Klumpke's paralysis paralysis of the forearm and hand caused by damage to the lower brachial nerve plexus. A birth injury often associated with excessive traction on the neck to assist the birth of the anterior shoulder.

knee–chest position a position assumed by the woman in which she rests on forearms and knees with hips elevated. Most often adopted when there is a cord presentation or prolapse, or where there is a need to encourage the presenting part out of the pelvis.

knee presentation a variation of breech presentation in which one or both knees of the fetus precede the buttocks.

'Know Your Midwife' scheme the model of care originally offered by a team of midwives in London as a pilot study to discover the advantages and disadvantages of the scheme and to be a model for future teams. Now commonly known as midwifery continuity of care.

Kocher's forceps surgical forceps with serrated jaws and sharp interlocking teeth at the lips. Occasionally used to artificially rupture the fetal membranes.

Koplik's spots white spots inside the mouth—the first sign of measles infection.

Korotkoff method a means of determining the diastolic blood pressure reading. There are five Korotkoff sounds distinguishable as the diastolic sound diminishes. Health professionals should note which sound they record as it makes a difference to the diagnosis of hypertension in pregnancy.

Krukenberg's tumour bilateral metastatic carcinoma of the ovaries, usually secondary to gastric carcinoma.

kwashiorkor a form of malnutrition that occurs after severe protein deficiency.

kyphosis convex, deformed curvature of the spine resulting in a hump on the back.

labia (SINGULAR labium) the two fleshy folds of skin on either side of the opening to the vagina. Labia majora are the outer fleshy folds; labia minora are the inner skin folds.

labial referring to the labia.

labile unstable, not fixed, subject to variations. Will change to different values at different times.

labour (SYNONYM parturition, childbirth) the process of giving birth. Artificially divided into three stages. The first stage of labour refers to the dilation of the cervical os to 10 cm. The second stage is from the full dilation of the cervical os to the complete birth of the baby. The third stage of labour refers to the expulsion of the placenta and membranes.

Labour Care Guide (LCG) a tool developed by the World Health Organization that aims to support good-quality, evidence-based, respectful care during labour and childbirth, irrespective of the setting or level of healthcare.

laboured breathing respiration which is difficult, noisy and uses all ancillary respiratory muscles. Present in preterm neonates with respiratory distress syndrome.

laceration a tear or injury.

lacrimal referring to the tears. The *lacrimal ducts* are part of the drainage system that carries tears from the *lacrimal glands*, the tear-secreting glands, to the nose.

lactalbumin the most important protein in human breast milk.

lactase an enzyme produced by the small intestine which splits lactose into monosaccharides and galactose.

lactation the secretion of milk by the breasts.

lacteals the lymphatic vessels surrounding the intestines which absorb split fats.

lactic acid an acid which is formed when there is a reduction in the amount of oxygen available for use in the body (hypoxic episodes). It causes the blood to become more acid (acidaemia). It is also found in the vagina and is produced by the action of bacilli on lactose. The acid climate created protects against some pathogenic organisms.

lactiferous conveying milk.

Lactobacillus acidophilus (SYNONYM Döderlein's bacillus) bacteria which grow in the vagina and convert glycogen to lactic acid which is said to prevent the growth of other organisms. It is also found in the stools of breastfed babies and has the same function.

lactoferrin the iron-binding protein found in human milk. It protects the infant from infection caused by the *E. coli* bacterium.

lactogen a substance which enables lactation. *Human placental lactogen* is a hormone secreted by the placenta which promotes growth and inhibits insulin's activity during pregnancy.

lactoglobulin a protein found in milk.

lactose a sugar found in milk. *Lactose intolerance* occurs when there is not enough lactase to split the sugar so it can be absorbed for use in the body. The condition causes diarrhoea and faltering growth and is treated by giving lactose-free milk.

lactulose a mild medicine given by mouth to treat constipation; it may take up to 48 hours to be effective.

laked describes blood that has haemolysed (erythrocytes which have split into their iron and protein components) due to severe infection, poisoning or burns.

Lamaze method preparation for childbirth developed by a French obstetrician based on a psychoprophylactic technique for changing the brain's perception of pain.

lambda sign seen by ultrasound as a thickened area of placental tissue at the site of insertion of the separating membranes suggesting a dichorionic placentation and non-identical twins.

lambda the posterior fontanelle which may be felt at the back of the fetal skull.

lambdoidal suture the crease felt at the side of the fetal skull running between the occipital bone and the parietal bone.

lamellar exfoliation of the newborn a congenital abnormality in which the infant is born with a scaly membrane over the skin. It peels off within 48 hours of birth.

lancet a short, pointed blade used to obtain a drop of blood for a capillary sample.

Langerhans islets *see* islets of Langerhans.

Langhans' cell layer the inside layer of the trophoblast.

lanolin the fat on (mainly) sheep's wool which is the basis for ointments.

lanugo the fine hair which covers the fetus in utero and is shed into the liquor just before term.

laparoscopic sterilisation a surgical procedure in which clips are applied to the fallopian tubes through a small incision in the abdomen. The sperm's passage towards the ovum is blocked, thereby preventing pregnancy.

laparotomy an opening made into a body cavity to examine the contents.

large for gestational age a baby whose growth is greater than the 90th centile. May be caused by genetic factors or maternal diabetes.

laryngoscope an instrument used to inspect the larynx and vocal cords. It aids insertion of an endotracheal tube which gives access to the lungs.

larynx the voice box, part of the air passages situated between the trachea and the base of the tongue.

last menstrual period (LMP) the date of the first day of the last normal menses. It is used to calculate the estimated date of birth of a baby using Nägele's rule.

late neonatal death death of a live-born baby after 7 completed days and before 28 completed days.

latent hidden.

latent activity changes which are happening but are not apparent, e.g. in the very early stages of labour.

latent phase the first stage of labour is a period of time characterised by painful uterine contractions and variable changes of the cervix, including some degree of effacement and slower progression of dilatation up to 5 cm.

late-onset Group B streptococcal disease neonatal infection that occurs after the first 7 days of life (see Group B streptococcal bacteria).

lateral referring to the side.

latex the sap of certain plants containing resins, proteins and other substances used to make rubber. It can cause allergic reactions in some individuals.

lavage washing out a cavity.

lavender oil an oil made from lavender flowers which has therapeutic properties.

laxative a mild medicine which promotes bowel evacuation by increasing the bulk of the faeces, softening the stool or lubricating the intestinal walls.

Leboyer method a very calm, quiet, darkened, warm environment is created around the birth of the baby. Leboyer, a French obstetrician, considered that this minimised the trauma of birth for both parents and child thereby creating greater satisfaction with the process.

lecithin a molecule made of a protein and a fat which is found in the alveoli of the lungs. It acts as a surfactant, which helps to keep the lungs open. The amount of this substance can be measured in amniotic fluid as an indicator of fetal maturity and likelihood of respiratory distress syndrome developing after delivery.

Lee-Frankenhauser plexus a network of nerves serving the cervix and pelvic cavity region of the body.

lesbian a term used when discussing sexual orientation. An individual who identifies as a woman and is romantically and/or sexually attracted to others who identify as women.

lesion 1. an injury or wound to a part of the body. 2. any structural abnormality or pathologic change in tissues.

'let-down' reflex neurogenic process which stimulates the release of milk from the breasts.

leucocyte (leukocyte) *see* leucocyte.

leucorrhoea (leukorrhoea) a white mucoid, inoffensive vaginal discharge. The amount is increased in pregnancy, at ovulation and during sexual arousal.

leucocyte (leukocyte) a white blood corpuscle (cell).

levator a strong muscle which raises and supports.

levator ani three muscles which stretch across the pelvic floor (see Fig. 53). They are the main support of the abdominal and pelvic organs.

LGBTQIA+ umbrella term that is used to refer to the community as a whole specifically referring to lesbian, gay, bisexual, transgender, queer, intersex, asexual and questioning communities to ensure inclusion and respect.

liability something one is obligated to do, or for which one must be accountable; an obligation under law, a responsibility.

libido desire for sexual intercourse.

lichen sclerosis atrophy and shrinkage of the skin of the vagina and vulva often accompanied by a chronic inflammatory reaction in the deeper tissues. Previously called kraurosis vulvae.

lie the relationship of the long axis of the fetus (spine) to the long axis of the woman's uterus. When they are parallel the lie is said to be longitudinal; when the fetal spine is across the mother's spine, the lie is transverse; and when the fetus is diagonal to the mother's spine the lie is oblique (see Fig. 54).

ligament a tough band of fibrous tissue connecting bones together or supporting organs.

ligature a thread (catgut, Vicryl or nylon) used for tying off

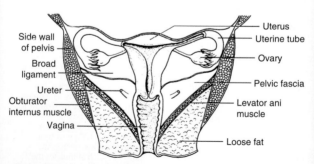

Figure 53
Levator ani

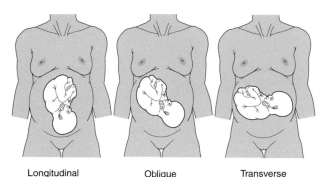

Longitudinal   Oblique   Transverse

Figure 54
Lie—longitudinal, oblique, transverse

blood vessels so they do not bleed.

light for dates *see* small for gestational age.

lightening the sensation experienced by women in late pregnancy when the fetus settles lower in the pelvis leaving more space in the upper abdomen.

linea alba the middle line of the abdomen representing the fusion of three strong sheets of fibrous tissue which cover the front of the abdomen.

linea nigra the pigmented line which appears during pregnancy, developing from the symphysis pubis upwards. The line fades slowly after pregnancy.

liquid based cytology (LBC) used in relation to cervical screening, this is a technique for taking and preparing slides to be read. Collected cervical cells are placed in a preservative liquid prior to testing. Largely replaces smearing cells on a slide (PAP smear test).

liquor (liquor amnii, SYNONYM amniotic fluid) the fluid which surrounds the fetus and fills out the uterine cavity. It is thought to be secreted by the fetal membranes lining the uterus. It is 99% water, with some proteins, fats and carbohydrates, fetal urine, lanugo, vernix and dead fetal cells. It allows growth and movement, acts as a shock absorber and equalises pressure on the fetus and placenta. There is approximately 1 litre at 37 weeks for an average-sized fetus but this decreases towards term.

listeria a gram-negative bacterium which causes upper respiratory infection, septicaemia and encephalitic disease.

lithopaedion a fetus who died in utero and became petrified; also called calcified fetus.

lithotomy position the woman lies on her back with her legs flexed, abducted and supported around two lithotomy poles in stirrups. The woman's legs must be lifted together by one person on each side of the bed because the hip joints are very soft due to the hormones in pregnancy and damage can easily occur.

litmus paper thin strips of blotting paper impregnated with the litmus pigment. It is used to find out if fluids are acid or alkaline. Blue litmus is turned red by acids and red litmus is turned blue by alkalis.

litre a measure of volume, 1000 mL.

live birth the complete expulsion or extraction from its mother of a product of conception, irrespective of the duration of the pregnancy, which, after such separation, the baby breathes or shows any other evidence of life, such as beating of the heart, pulsation of the umbilical cord, or definite movement of voluntary muscles, whether or not the umbilical cord has been cut or the placenta is attached; each product of such a birth is considered live-born.

liver the vital organ situated on the right side of the abdomen slightly under and protected by the ribs. It stores carbohydrates, iron and vitamins; destroys toxins, drugs, alcohol and poisons; makes bile, plasma proteins, antibodies, clotting factors (prothrombin and fibrinogen) and heat.

living guidelines approach an evidence-informed, consultative prioritisation process, rapid updating of prioritised systematic reviews and electronic consultations with 'living guidelines' panels.

living systematic review a process of active monitoring of the evidence to immediately include new evidence in reviews and recommendations.

lobe a section or small part of an organ separated from other parts by fibrous tissue or fissures.

lobule a small lobe or smaller section or segment of a lobe.

local anaesthesia a drug injected into tissue to reduce sensation in the area, e.g. as used before repair of the perineum.

local anaesthetic a drug given to prevent the transmission of impulses through nerves and stop sensation of pain registering in the brain, e.g. epidural anaesthetic.

lochia the vaginal loss after birth which is made up of blood, dead cells, liquor, vernix, meconium and other debris from the uterus. It changes over the first few days from *lochia rubra*, which is largely fresh blood, to *lochia serosa*, which is pink and contains more white than red blood cells, to *lochia alba*, which is whitish and mainly mucoid. These changes can take up to 3 or 4 weeks. Normal lochia changes progressively and does not smell offensive.

locked twins a rare condition where each twin is preventing the other from being born. Labour will be obstructed (*see* Fig. 55).

long COVID the name for the condition persisting after the typical recovery period after contracting COVID-19 disease.

long-acting removable contraception (LARC) contraceptives that are long lasting (3–5 years generally) and include intrauterine

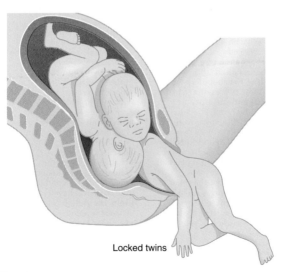

Locked twins

Figure 55
Locked twins

devices (IUDs) and hormonal implants.

longitudinal a measurement referring to the longest aspect of a body or organ.

longitudinal lie the long axis of the fetus (spine) is parallel to the long axis of the uterus. Presentation can be breech or cephalic.

lordosis a condition where the spine is curved more than the moderate degree seen in pregnancy. Normally the spine curves backwards as the body attempts to accommodate the extra abdominal weight and keep the centre of gravity over the feet. A degree of backache will be experienced.

Lövset's manoeuvre a technique used to assist the birth of the shoulders when the fetus is presenting by the breech and the arms are above the head. The fetus is rotated half a circle so that the posterior arm is twisted across the face and the elbow can be reached and delivered. The fetus is then rotated half a circle in the reverse direction so that the other arm can be born similarly.

low birth weight a baby weighing less than 2.5 kg either because it is preterm or because it is small for gestational age.

lower-segment caesarean section (LSCS) an operation during which the lower segment of the uterus is opened surgically from an abdominal wound in order for the baby to be born.

lower uterine segment the part of the uterus lying just above the cervix which will become relaxed, thin and incorporate the cervix during labour.

lubricant a cream or jelly applied to hands, gloves or instruments in order to make them slippery and easier to insert.

lumbar referring to the lower part of the spine.

lumbar puncture a diagnostic or treatment procedure during which a needle is introduced into the subarachnoid space and cerebrospinal fluid withdrawn or medication introduced (*see* Fig. 56).

lumen a space inside a tube.

lumpectomy surgical excision of only the palpable lesion in carcinoma of the breast.

lupus localised destruction or degeneration of the skin caused by various cutaneous diseases.

luteal referring to the corpus luteum on the outside of the ovary in the second half of the menstrual cycle.

lutein the yellow colour in the corpus luteum.

luteinising hormone a hormone secreted from the anterior part of the pituitary gland which with follicle-stimulating hormone causes ovulation and the formation of the corpus luteum in the female.

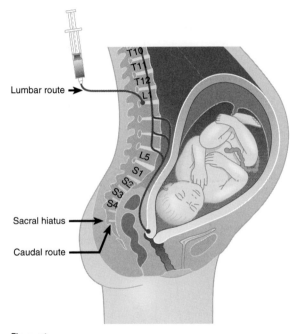

Figure 56
Lumbar puncture

In the male it promotes development of the interstitial cells and secretion of testosterone.

lying-in older, colloquial term for the specific period of time just before, during and after childbirth when a woman needs care and rest.

lymph exudate that surrounds the cells which drains into the *lymphatic system* (*see* Fig. 57) and then into the blood.

lymphatics the vessels which carry lymph.

lymphocyte white blood cells made in the bone marrow and thymus whose function is to fight infection.

lysis the gradual fall of a fever or breakdown of red blood cells.

lysozyme an antibacterial substance found in tissues, and secreted in tears and breast milk.

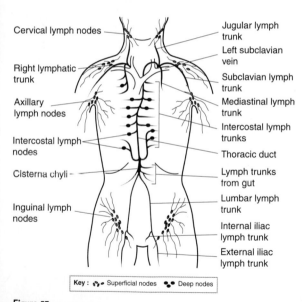

Cervical lymph nodes

Jugular lymph trunk

Left subclavian vein

Right lymphatic trunk

Subclavian lymph trunk

Axillary lymph nodes

Mediastinal lymph trunk

Intercostal lymph trunks

Intercostal lymph nodes

Thoracic duct

Cisterna chyli

Lymph trunks from gut

Inguinal lymph nodes

Lumbar lymph trunk

Internal iliac lymph trunk

External iliac lymph trunk

Key : ⚬⚬ Superficial nodes ●● Deep nodes

Figure 57
Lymphatic system

Mm

maceration the process of softening a solid mass by soaking it. A *macerated fetus* is an unborn baby who has died in utero and has been soaked in liquor so that it has become soft. Its skin is blue and peels, and it may disintegrate. This indicates that the baby has died before labour. Enzymes released from the tissue may cause a serious complication to the mother called disseminated intravascular coagulation (DIC).

Mackenrodt's ligament the transverse or cardinal ligament that supports the uterus at the cervical level within the pelvic cavity.

macrencephaly a large brain, which is usually a congenital condition.

macro- combining form meaning large.

macrocephaly a large head and brain in comparison to the rest of the body. Mental and physical impairment are usually present.

macrocyte an abnormally large red blood cell. Macrocytic erythrocytes are found in the blood in megaloblastic anaemia of pregnancy due to lack of folic acid in the diet during the cells' manufacture.

macrogenitosomia enlargement of the external genitalia

in boys and pseudohermaphroditism in girls. It is congenital in origin.

macroglossia enlargement of the tongue.

macrognathia enlargement of the jaw.

macroscopic visible with the naked eye.

macular rash many small, flat, red spots on the skin.

magnesium (Mg) an element essential for life.

magnesium sulfate a salt of magnesium prescribed intravenously to prevent seizures, especially in pre-eclampsia, and by mouth to treat constipation and heartburn (*magnesium trisilicate*). The latter may be given before general anaesthetic to reduce the acidity of the gastric contents and thereby prevent Mendelson's syndrome.

magnetic resonance imaging (MRI) the use of radio frequency radiation as a means of obtaining images of the internal parts of the body.

mal- combining form meaning bad, wrong or ill; a disorder. *Grand mal* is a generalised fit or convulsion; *petit mal* is a momentary loss of consciousness without convulsion.

malabsorption inability to absorb nutrients from the

intestines. The nutrients will be passed out in the stools (*malabsorption syndrome*).

malaise a feeling of general discomfort, loss of energy or illness.

malaria a tropical infection transmitted through the skin by a mosquito bite. The insect injects a protozoal parasite which develops in the erythrocyte causing anaemia, febrile illness and splenomegaly.

male refers to the sex that produces sperm cells and fertilises the female ovum (egg) in the process of reproduction.

malformation an anatomical abnormality, either acquired or congenital.

malignant a term applied to a condition which will become progressively degenerative and result in death.

malnutrition a disorder of the diet, either incorrect foods or not enough food.

malposition in the wrong place. Refers to a position of the fetus in the uterus which will not aid normal progress in labour (*see* Fig. 58).

malpractice inadequate skills, care or conduct from a professionally qualified person. It can result in injury,

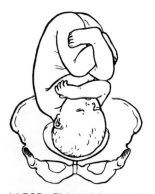

(a) ROP – Right occipito posterior

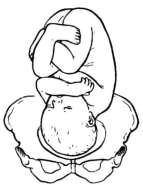

(b) LOP – left occipito posterior

Figure 58

Malposition (a) right occipitoposterior (ROP) (b) left occipitoposterior (LOP)

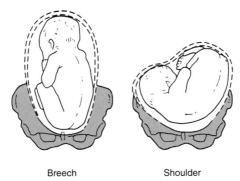

Breech   Shoulder

Figure 59
Malpresentation

suffering or death. Used in law to denote negligence (that which a reasonable person would not do).

malpresentation when the fetal head is not over the cervix; the breech, brow, shoulder or face may be found instead (*see* Fig. 59).

maltase an enzyme which splits maltose into glucose. Found in the pancreatic and intestinal juices.

maltose a sugar formed when starch is decomposed by the action of amylase.

mammary referring to the breasts.

mammillary referring to the nipples.

mammography X-ray examination of the breasts to look for cancers and other disorders. A contrast medium may be used.

mandelic acid a drug used as an antiseptic in the treatment of urinary tract infections including cystitis, nephritis and pyelitis.

mandible the lower jaw bone.

mania a severe mental disorder. Associated with rapid, extreme mood swings and possible violence.

manic-depressive psychosis (*see* bipolar disorder) a previous term for mental illness characterised by alternating attacks of mania and depression.

manipulation using the hands in a skilled manner to change a position, e.g. the fetus in the uterus or bones in the spine.

manoeuvre a procedure carried out with the hands, e.g. *Lövset's manoeuvre*.

manometer an instrument used to measure pressure or tension, e.g. of blood in the arteries.

Mantoux test a test to detect immunity to tuberculosis (TB). A small amount of old tuberculin is injected under the skin. A reaction indicates immunity.

manual with the hands.

manual handling the use of muscular force (or effort) to lift, move, push, pull, carry, hold or restrain any object, including a person. In health settings, care is taken to ensure that injuries to staff do not occur due to manual handling, especially assisting in the movement of patients.

manual removal of the placenta the removal of the placenta from the uterus by inserting a hand into the uterus and separating the placenta from the uterine wall (*see* Fig. 60).

manual rotation turning of the baby's head from a transverse position by internally applied

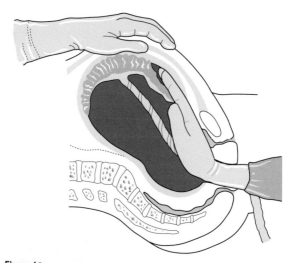

Figure 60
Manual removal of the placenta

pressure to dislodge its fixture on the ischial spines and rotating it to a more favourable position, that is, occipitoanterior or occipitoposterior.

maple syrup urine disease an inherited metabolic disorder where the enzyme necessary for the breakdown of the amino acids valine, leucine and isoleucine is absent. Infants or children may be identified as having the disorder due to the odour of their urine, mental and physical disability and hyperreflexia.

marasmus severe malnutrition and weight loss in babies and infants associated with protein and calorie deficiency.

Marfan's syndrome a hereditary condition recognised by elongation of the bones, often in association with abnormalities of the eyes and cardiovascular system.

marginal placenta praevia a placenta which is low-lying, its edges located on the margin of the lower segment of the uterus, possibly reaching the internal cervical os.

marijuana prepared from the hemp plant *Cannabis sativa*. Hashish is made from the flowers of the same plant. It is usually smoked but can be ingested. It gives a feeling of euphoria and may relieve pain. Possession and supply of marijuana in most places in Australia and New Zealand is illegal.

marrow the fatty, sponge-like material in the cavity of bones. It is responsible for the manufacture of all types of blood cells.

masculine having the characteristics and features of a male.

massage stroking or kneading of the body to aid relaxation, stimulate circulation and excretion, and lower blood pressure. In labour some women like to be stroked over the abdomen or kneaded over the lower spine. *Cardiac massage* is carried out when the heart stops, for the purpose of resuscitation; externally the heart is compressed between the ribs and the spine, or it can be done internally by hand following opening of the chest wall.

mast cell (SYNONYM mastocyte) a cell found in several types of tissues that contains granules that are rich in histamine and heparin. Mast cells are involved in allergies and anaphylaxis and are also important for wound healing.

mastalgia pain in the breast, for which there are a number of different causes.

mastectomy the excision of the breast, usually done to remove a malignant tumour.

mastitis inflammation of the breasts.

masturbation pleasurable stimulation of the genitals by oneself or with a partner (*mutual masturbation*), often to the point of orgasm.

materia medica the study of drugs—sources, preparations, uses and effects. *Homeopathic materia medica* is the study of homeopathic remedies which have been tested on human volunteers.

maternal referring to the mother; the quality of being a mother.

maternal antibodies antibodies transferred from the mother to the baby across the placenta. Babies are born with some immunity.

maternal death the death of the mother during pregnancy, labour and birth and the first 42 days after the birth. Deaths are defined as direct, indirect and incidental. Late deaths can also be counted up to 12 months after the birth.

maternal-infant bonding the complex process by which the mother and child become emotionally attached. It starts during pregnancy and may take some time to accomplish. Interaction and responsiveness are shared.

maternal mortality ratio (MMR) defined by the World Health Organization as the number of (direct and indirect) maternal deaths over the number of women who gave birth during a time period.

maternity motherhood.

matrix an intercellular substance, the basic building block from which a specific organ or kind of tissue develops.

Matthews-Duncan expulsion of the placenta the maternal surface of the placenta is seen first at the vulva during the third stage of labour (*see* Fig. 61). The cause may be a lower-lying placenta. (*Compare* Schultze expulsion.)

maturation the process by which the greatest possible amount of development is achieved.

mature fully developed, having ripened, reached full potential.

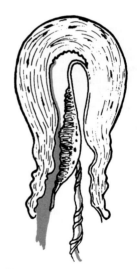

Figure 61
Matthews-Duncan expulsion of the placenta

Mauriceau-Smellie-Veit manoeuvre a method of assisting the birth of the aftercoming head when a vaginal breech birth is occurring. Flexion of the head is promoted and jaw and shoulder traction is applied by the hands of the operator who has one hand over the shoulders with the middle finger on the occiput, and the other hand over the chest with the middle finger on the jaw bone. The modified Mauriceau–Smellie–Veit manoeuvre is now recommended which involves two fingers on the malar prominences rather than the jaw to reduce the risk of jaw dislocation.

mean one form of measurement of central tendency; all the values in a group are added together and divided by the number of values to reach the mean or average.

measles a highly infectious disease caused by a virus. Mortality rate is high in some parts of the world. Routine immunisation is given after the infant is 1 year old.

measles, mumps and rubella vaccine (MMR) an active immunising agent prescribed to protect the child (or an adult) against these diseases. It is given after the first year of life.

meatus an anatomical passageway opening into or out of an organ.

mechanism of labour a sequence of movements made by the baby as it adapts itself to the changing dimensions of the pelvis during the second stage of labour.

meconium sticky green/black material passed by the baby during the first couple of days after birth. It contains bile pigments, salts, mucus and cells which have collected during pregnancy. It may be passed in utero, as a result of fetal stress or during periods of hypoxia (also called meconium-stained liquor).

meconium aspiration inhalation of meconium-contaminated liquor causing damage to the lining of the lungs.

meconium plug syndrome the meconium becomes very thick and causes the large intestine to be obstructed. The newborn infant will not pass meconium, will have a distended bowel and may vomit.

median 1. situated in the middle or midline. 2. a form of measurement of central tendency where a number of values are placed in order (e.g. from least to greatest) and the central one is taken as the median average.

median nerve the nerve that extends along the radial parts of the forearm and the hand. Can be damaged in shoulder dystocia or in some breech births where the baby's arm needs to be manually released.

mediastinum the space containing the lungs behind the sternum and in between the two pleural sacs.

medical abortion a means to end an unwanted pregnancy using two medications: mifepristone and misoprostol. Together the medications weaken the attachment of the pregnancy to the uterus and also cause the uterus to contract causing bleeding to expel the pregnancy This procedure can be undertaken up to 9 weeks of pregnancy. Medical abortion is not legal in many countries.

MEDLARS an acronym for Medical Literature Analysis and Retrieval System, a computerised bibliographic system from which the Index Medicus is produced.

MEDLINE an acronym for MEDLARS Online.

medulla the central or inside region of an organ. The *medulla oblongata* is the lowest part of the brain at the back just before the spine starts. It controls the vital centres, heart, respiration, etc.

mega- combining form meaning large or as a prefix meaning million, as in megawatt, megavolt, etc.

megaloblastic anaemia an anaemia associated with pregnancy in which the red blood cells are large and immature and therefore do not bind with oxygen. It is caused by a folic acid deficiency and treated with the same.

megaloblasts large immature red blood cells found in the bone marrow which nevertheless have a nucleus.

meiosis the division of the sex cell into two haploid gametes, the nucleus of each receiving half the number of chromosomes (23).

melaena the passage of dark and pitchy stools stained with blood pigments or with altered blood.

melanin the black or dark brown pigment which occurs naturally in skin, hair and the iris of the eye. In pregnancy there is an increase in the pigmentation giving rise to the linea nigra, darkened areolas and sometimes chloasma.

membrane a thin tissue covering organs and lining cavities. Frequently responsible for secreting mucus or hormones. Fetal membranes are the amnion and the chorion.

membrane strip a procedure performed during vaginal examination, where a finger is inserted through the external cervical os and gently frees the membranes from the wall of the lower segment of the uterus. This may stimulate the release of oxytocin and commencement of labour.

menarche the onset of menstruation; the first menstrual period.

Mendel's law the principles of genetic inheritance which indicate how characteristics are passed from one generation to the next.

Mendelson's syndrome an inflammatory response to inhalation of regurgitated gastric juices during the induction of a general anaesthetic. The juices burn the lining of the lungs causing irritation, spasm and oedema. Can occasionally be fatal, but is preventable by the application of cricoid pressure.

meninges the three membranes covering the brain and spinal cord: dura mater, arachnoid mater and pia mater.

meningitis inflammation of the meninges characterised by headaches, stiffness of the neck, irritability, malaise, nausea, vomiting, delirium, pyrexia and tachycardia. Can be fatal.

meningocele a congenital abnormality characterised by a defect in the skull or vertebral column through which the meninges protrude. The sac is filled with cerebrospinal fluid (*see* Fig. 62).

meningoencephalocele a hernia-like protrusion of meninges and brain tissue through a defect in the skull.

meningomyelocele a hernia-like protrusion of meninges and spinal cord through a defect in the vertebral column (*see* Fig. 63).

menopause the normal, permanent cessation of menstruation. It signifies the end of the reproductive phase of a woman's life.

menorrhagia unusually heavy bleeding during menstruation.

menorrhoea normal discharge of blood and tissue from the uterus once a month; menstruation.

menostasis impediment in the menstrual flow—discharges cannot escape from the uterus or vagina owing to an occlusion.

menses menstruation.

menstrual referring to menstruation, as in *menstrual period*, the period during the menstrual cycle in which menstruation occurs.

menstrual age (SYNONYM gestational age) the age of an embryo or fetus is calculated from the first day of the last normal menstrual period.

menstrual cycle the recurring cycle of changes in the endometrium of the uterus (*see* Fig. 64). The decidual layer grows, proliferates, is maintained for several days and then shed at the next period, usually 28 days later. The cycle is controlled by hormones from the pituitary gland and from the ovaries. The duration and length of the cycle varies greatly among women. This cyclical process begins at the menarche and ends at the menopause.

menstruation (SYNONYM menses, menstrual period) the shedding of blood, cells and other debris from the degenerated deciduas which

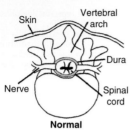

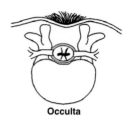

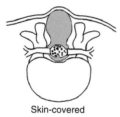

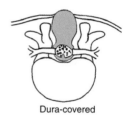

Figure 62
Meningocele

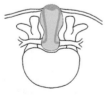

Figure 63
Meningomyelocele

pass from the non-pregnant uterus through the vagina. It happens at approximately 28-day intervals and lasts about 4–5 days, although there are wide variations in these averages between individual women.

mental pertaining to the mind.

mentoanterior the position of the fetus in the uterus with the chin at the front of the pelvis (*see* Fig. 65). Other possible chin positions are

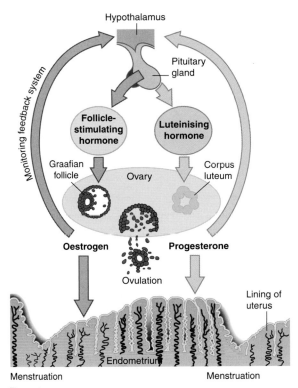

Figure 64
Menstrual cycle

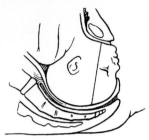

Figure 65
Mentoanterior

mentoposterior and mentolateral.

mentor an experienced practitioner who helps or guides a student or less experienced person.

mentum the chin; used as the denominator in a face presentation of the fetus.

MEOWS *see* modified early obstetric warning score or system.

meridian one of the energy lines running throughout the body along which acupuncture points are located in traditional Chinese medicine.

MERS *see* Middle East Respiratory Syndrome.

mesentery the membranes which line the abdominal cavity and fold over to hold the abdominal organs in place.

mesoderm the layer of cells between the ectoderm and the endoderm in the embryo which will develop into bone, muscle, heart, blood, gonads, kidneys and connective tissue.

mesosalpinx the part of the peritoneum which covers the fallopian tubes.

mesovarium the part of the peritoneum connecting the ovary to the broad ligament.

meta-analysis combines the results of several studies that address a set of related research hypotheses. This is the statistical technique used in systematic reviews.

metabolic acidosis an abnormal physiological state in which there is excessive loss of bicarbonate from the body and accumulation of acids in the blood.

metabolism all the processes that take place in living organisms resulting in growth, energy, elimination and other bodily functions as they relate to the use of nutrients in the blood after absorption from the gut.

metastasis the transfer of disease from one organ or part to another not directly connected with it. A cancer resulting from the spread of the primary tumour.

metatarsus the part of the foot between ankle and toes where there are five metatarsals.

methadone hydrochloride a synthetic compound with effects similar to that of morphine and heroin. Prescribed in pregnancy to drug-dependent women as a maintenance drug.

metra-, metro- prefix meaning uterus.

metralgia tenderness or pain in the uterus.

metre (m) the fundamental unit of length in the International System of Units (SI).

metric system a decimalised system of measurement based on kilograms, metres and litres rather than pounds, feet and pints.

metritis inflammation of the walls of the uterus; may be *endometritis* or *parametritis*.

metropathia haemorrhagica excessive painless menstrual and intermenstrual bleeding accompanied by lack of ovulation.

metroplasty surgical operation to repair the uterus.

metrorrhagia bleeding from the uterus that is not the menstrual period.

metrostaxis persistent slight bleeding from the uterus

micro- combining form meaning very small.

microbe an organism too small to see with the naked eye. Can be seen with a microscope.

microcephaly abnormal smallness of the head. Such babies are mentally subnormal.

microgenitalism abnormal smallness of the external reproductive organs.

micrognathia abnormal smallness of the lower jaw bone; receding chin. Associated with Pierre Robin syndrome.

micron one millionth part of a metre—a micrometre.

microorganism a tiny living cell too small to be seen with the human eye.

microphage a neutrophil capable of ingesting small organisms such as bacteria.

micturition passing of urine.

Middle East respiratory syndrome (MERS) a viral respiratory disease caused by a novel coronavirus (MERS-CoV)

midstream urine, midstream catch urine specimen a collection of urine obtained after the genitalia have been cleansed, the stream started, the mid-section saved and voiding completed in the toilet. It should be freer from contamination than a standard urine sample.

mid-upper arm circumference (MUAC) is a useful tool for a fast assessment of the nutritional status. It is an easy and inexpensive way to detect nutritional status and is used in low-income countries for rapid and extensive nutrition surveillance and screening programs.

midwife traditionally, a woman who was with other women during childbirth. The international definition states that 'a midwife is a person who has successfully completed a midwifery education program that is duly recognised in the country where it is located and that is based on the International Confederation of Midwives (ICM) Essential Competencies for Midwifery Practice and the framework of the ICM Global Standards for Midwifery Education; who has acquired the requisite qualifications to be registered and/or legally licensed to practice midwifery and use the title "midwife"; and who demonstrates competency in the practice of midwifery' (ICM International Definition of the Midwife 2011).

midwifery the art and science concerned with caring for women and their families during normal pregnancy, labour and the postnatal period.

midwifery group practice small groups of midwives (usually four to six; often working in pairs) who provide all antenatal, intrapartum and postnatal midwifery care for a defined number of women.

milia neonatorum tiny cysts found on the face or trunk of the newborn.

military attitude used to describe the fetal head which is neither flexed nor deflexed.

milk the bodily fluid secreted by the mammary glands.

milk bank a stored supply of human milk for future use by other individuals. The World Health Organization and UNICEF support donor mothers' milk as the first alternative where mother's milk is not available.

milk ejection reflex (SYNONYM 'let-down' reflex) as the baby starts sucking at the breast the neurohormonal arch is stimulated and oxytocin is released from the posterior aspect of the pituitary gland. It causes the myoepithelial cells to contract forcing the milk towards the nipple.

milk fever the mild pyrexia occurring on postnatal days 4 and 5 as lactation commences.

milli- a prefix meaning one-thousandth of the whole, e.g. milligram (mg), millilitre (mL), millimetre (mm).

miscarriage (SYNONYM abortion) the spontaneous loss from the uterus of a baby before the 20th week of gestation. It may be loss altogether (*complete abortion*) or in part (*incomplete abortion*) or the fetus may die and be retained (*missed abortion*).

misoprostol medication used to start labour, cause a termination of pregnancy, prevent and treat stomach ulcers, and treat postpartum bleeding due to poor contraction of the uterus.

mitosis the way in which cells reproduce themselves. The nucleus divides and so does each chromosome so that two identical cells are produced.

mittelschmerz pain between menstrual periods; thought to originate in the reproductive organs and to coincide with ovulation.

mode a measurement of central tendency which comprises the value or term which occurs more frequently than any other value or term.

modified early obstetric warning score or system (MEOWS) an observation chart developed to assist clinicians with early recognition of clinical deterioration through the monitoring and scoring of physical parameters such as blood pressure, heart rate and respirations. The scoring system provides levels of alert and when to seek clinical review.

module a short program of study in a specific area designed to meet a limited number of objectives. Modules can be awarded credit towards a higher qualification.

molar pregnancy a hydatidiform mole develops after conception instead of a fetus. All the signs of pregnancy are severely exaggerated. Removal under anaesthetic is usually required.

mole 1. in dermatology, a small area of skin which is deeply pigmented. 2. in obstetrics, a hydatidiform mole. 3. in science, a unit of measure of a substance.

molecular genetics the branch of genetic study which focuses on the chemical transmission of information, that is, deoxyribonucleic acid (DNA).

molecule the smallest particle of a substance or fluid. Molecules are different sizes depending on the material of which they form a part. Molecules contain atoms.

Mongolian blue spot a smooth brown or greyish area of skin present at birth. It is due to an excess of melanocytes in one particular area, frequently over the sacrum. They fade or disappear during childhood.

mongolism an obsolete term for Down syndrome.

monitrice a labour assistant, usually a person with special training in the Lamaze method of childbirth.

monoamine oxidase inhibitors (MAOI) a group of drugs used to treat depression.

monosaccharide the simplest form of sugar.

monotropy a mother's ability to bond with only one child of twins at a time.

monozygote referring to, or developed from, a single fertilised cell. The cell divides and identical twins can develop (*see* Fig. 66).

mons veneris the area over the symphysis pubis which is covered with hair.

Montgomery's glands, Montgomery's tubercles sebaceous glands around the nipples which secrete a lubricating substance that protects the nipple from infection and trauma during breastfeeding.

morbid diseased, physically or mentally.

morbidity the condition of being diseased.

morbidity rate the number of cases of a particular disease occurring in a year in a specific number of the population. It may be calculated on the basis of age group, live or stillbirth, sex or other population unit.

'morning after' pill a large dose of oestrogen given orally within 72 hours of unprotected sexual intercourse to prevent a conception occurring.

morning sickness the feeling of nausea and occasional vomiting sometimes associated

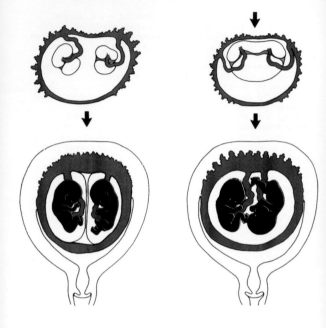

(a) Separate amnions;
    common chorion
    and placenta

(b) Common amnion
    chorion and placenta

Figure 66
Monozygotic twins

with early pregnancy. It may
happen at any time of day.
Moro reflex the response of a
healthy newborn baby to a
sudden noise or the falling
back of its head. The arms
swing out and return to a
central position in a series of
small jerks.
morphine sulfate a powerful
drug made from opium given
on a doctor's prescription to

relieve severe pain. It may cause depression of the respiratory centre in the brain.

mortality rate (SYNONYM death rate) the number of deaths in a given population, e.g. *maternal, neonatal* or *infant mortality rate.*

morula the fertilised ovum at 4 days old, when cell division has occurred and it resembles a small mulberry.

motile sperm organelle morphology examination (MSOME) assessing sperm shape under very high magnification.

motor nerves the nerves through which impulses pass from the spinal cord to muscles instructing them to move in a desired manner.

moulding a process of alteration of the shape and size of the fetal head during its passage through the maternal pelvis as it accommodates itself to the bony structure while protecting the brain (*see* Fig. 67). The soft sutures between the bones allow overriding of the bones and this can be felt on vaginal examination.

mouth-to-mouth resuscitation a procedure in which the mouth of a breathing person covers that of a non-breathing person and air is forcibly blown into the non-breathing lungs to maintain oxygenation and so maintain the person's life.

movements *fetal movements* start as twitches and progress

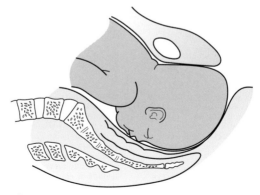

Figure 67
Moulding

to full limb and breathing movements. The woman is usually aware of them from 16–19 weeks' gestation.

mucoid describes a body fluid as being thick and like egg white.

mucopurulent containing mucus which is infected and yellowed by the presence of pus.

mucosa *see* mucous membrane.

mucous referring to or secreting mucus.

mucous membrane (SYNONYM mucosa) a thin sheet of tissue which covers or lines cavities, organs and canals in the body. Its function is to protect structures, secrete mucus to prevent friction and allow movement, and absorb water, salts and other substances (including drugs).

mucus a clear, thick fluid secreted by the body to reduce friction between adjacent tissues.

mucus plug the operculum is the plug of mucus which fills the cervical canal during pregnancy and is shed as the 'show' at the commencement of cervical dilation in labour. It prevents the entry of sperm and most microorganisms.

müllerian ducts the ducts present in early fetal life which in females will fuse to become the vagina, uterus and fallopian tubes. Most of the ducts will disappear in the male fetus.

multicultural refers to a community in which people

from many different cultures and ethnic backgrounds live.

multidisciplinary team a group of people each educated in a specific and different branch of healthcare who work together to achieve common objectives.

multifactorial a situation in which many factors will be relevant and influence the result.

multigravida a pregnant woman who has had at least one previous pregnancy.

multipara a woman who has given birth to more than one infant.

multiple pregnancy a pregnancy in which there is more than one fetus in the uterus. Twins occur spontaneously in approximately 1 in every 80 pregnancies. Triplet and higher-order pregnancies are less common.

multiple sclerosis a progressive disease in which nerves become demyelinated giving rise to strange sensations and symptoms of ataxia, tremor and urogenital disturbances among others.

mumps a communicable disease caused by a virus infecting the parotid glands (saliva-producing glands in the mouth).

murmur a sound heard periodically on auscultation, usually of cardiac or vascular origin. It is deemed pathological.

muscle a specialised group of cells with the ability to

contract and relax. The cells may be arranged in bundles and pairs will work opposite each other in the major limbs. They may be arranged in circular formation and called sphincters, e.g. the anus and the iris, or they may be arranged in sheets and not be under the control of the central nervous system, as in the intestines.

muscular dystrophy a genetic disease in which generalised muscle wasting occurs resulting in crippling. Duchenne muscular dystrophy is a sex-linked recessive disease in which a woman carries the gene and will pass it on to her daughters, who may become carriers, or her sons, one in two of whom will inherit the condition. It can now be detected antenatally by DNA studies.

mutation a change in form, quality or some other characteristic.

myasthenia muscular debility; any constitutional anomaly of muscle.

myocardium the middle and thickest layer of the heart wall, composed of cardiac muscle.

myoepithelial cells epithelial cells that can contract like smooth muscle cells. They are present in glands, notably the mammary gland which enables breastfeeding to occur.

myoma a tumour composed of muscle tissue.

myomectomy the removal of fibroids (non-cancerous tumours) from the wall of the uterus.

myometrium the uterine muscle.

myxoedema a condition associated with hypothyroidism (primary myxoedema) or hypopituitarism (secondary or pituitary myxoedema). Characteristics include dry hair and skin, thickened skin of the lips and puffy eyelids.

Nn

Naboth's cysts (nabothian cysts) small cysts on the cervix caused by blockage of the entrance to the nabothian glands.

nabothian glands mucus-secreting glands on the uterine cervix.

NAD acronym meaning nothing abnormal detected.

naevus (nevus) a birthmark caused by a small area of dilated capillary blood vessels on the skin.

Nägele's pelvis a pelvis in which one of the sacral ala fails to develop causing the pelvis to be abnormally shaped and making a normal birth difficult.

Nägele's rule a method of calculating the expected date of birth of the fetus. Subtract 3 months from the date of the first day of the last normal menstrual period and add a year and 7 days, or add 7 days and 9 months to the date of the last normal menstrual period. This system presumes a 28-day menstrual cycle and has been shown to be less than optimally accurate.

nano- prefix meaning one thousand millionth, e.g. *nanogram* (ng).

nappy rash occurs on the area covered by a baby's nappy. There are red areas, which may have tiny raised patches resembling blisters. It can be caused by the skin being covered or enclosed, ammonia in the urine being in contact with the skin for a long time, or by fungal infection.

narco- combining form meaning stupor.

narcosis a reversible condition marked by stupor or insensibility, produced by opioid drugs and certain other substances.

narcotic a drug which lowers the conscious level to produce insensibility or stupor.

narcotic addiction a habit of taking narcotic drugs.

narcotic antagonist a drug used to reverse the respiratory-depressing effect of narcotic drugs.

nares the nostrils.

nasal relating to the nose.

nasogastric tube a thin, soft latex tube passed into the stomach via the nose in order to assess patency of the oesophagus, to aspirate mucus or to feed.

nasojejunal feeding a method in which a silicone-coated catheter is passed through the nose into the jejunum, to provide nutrition to the baby.

nasopharynx that part of the nose above the soft palate of the mouth.

natal referring to birth.

natural childbirth a philosophy which encourages giving birth without routine medical intervention.

natural family planning controlling fertility without resort to medication or mechanical devices, the principle being to avoid unprotected intercourse around the time of ovulation as predicted by measuring basal temperature, checking physical signs such as cervical position and quality of mucus or calculating likely ovulation date from data on previous cycles.

nausea the sensation of wanting to be sick.

navel the umbilicus or belly button.

NBAC next birth after caesarean.

necro- combining form meaning death.

necrosis death of a small mass of tissue within a larger mass as a result of injury or infection.

necrotic affected by necrosis.

necrotising enterocolitis inflammation of the gut wall of a neonate as a result of infection. Recognised by acute abdominal pain, blood in the stools and vomiting, the condition may lead to septicaemia and is life-threatening.

needlestick injury accidental damage to the skin of a person by a needle which has previously been used to treat another person.

neglected tropical diseases (NTDs) diseases that generally afflict the poorest countries and historically have not received as much attention as other diseases. Examples of NTDs include dengue, trachoma, leprosy and soil-transmitted helminths (intestinal worms).

negligence a deficiency in the care delivered as compared to that delivered by a reasonable person in the same circumstances. If damage results it is a professional offence and will be investigated and disciplined within the profession as authorised by legislation. Victims of negligence may seek legal advice regarding compensation.

nem a nutritional unit described as 1 g of breast milk of specific nutritional components having a caloric value equivalent to 2/3 calorie.

neo- combining form meaning new, young.

neonatal pertaining to the newborn infant from birth up to 4 weeks of age.

neonatal abstinence syndrome (SYNONYM neonatal withdrawal syndrome) a defined set of behavioural and physiological signs and symptoms common to babies whose mothers used drugs of addiction during pregnancy.

Neonatal Behavioural Assessment Scale (NBAS) a means of assessing an infant's condition, alertness, motor function, irritability, consolability and interaction with people.

neonatal death (NND) death of a live-born baby within 28 days of birth.

neonatal morbidity any condition or disease of the baby that occurs in the neonatal period.

neonatal mortality rate the number of deaths among infants 28 days old, per 1000 live births occurring within 1 year.

neonatal period the time from birth until 28 days of age when the infant is at greatest risk of infection and faltering growth.

neonatal thermoregulation newborn babies are incapable of achieving a balance of heat loss and heat retention. They lose heat through conduction, radiation, evaporation and convection. Care is required to minimise heat loss by drying and covering the baby (especially the head) quickly after birth.

neonatal unit an area of a hospital especially resourced and staffed to meet the needs of babies born unwell, premature or with injuries and abnormalities.

neonate a newborn baby during its first 28 days of life.

neonatology the study, treatment and care of neonates.

NeoPuff manually controlled infant resuscitator (like an automated bag and mask) which delivers breaths manually with accurate peak inspiratory pressure (PIP) and positive-end expiratory pressure (PEEP).

nephritis inflammation of a kidney. It is usually secondary to an infection somewhere else in the body.

nephron a unit of the kidney's substance which is involved in filtration of blood.

nerve a fibre which carries messages between the brain and the different parts of the body.

nerve block disruption of the neural pathway by drugs. Sensation of pain is interrupted by nerves being bathed in a drug such as bupivacaine. Otherwise known as epidural analgesia.

nervous system the channels supplying the whole body which transmit to the brain (control centre) information about the environment. The channels contain nerves (peripheral nerves) which enter and leave the spinal cord through which their information is relayed to the brain.

network socially and professionally, a range of people with whom one has some things in common and from whom one could seek help and advice if required.

neural tube defect (NTD) when the bones do not grow over the spinal column completely during early fetal development thereby allowing exposure or protrusion of part of the central nervous system, as in open or occult spina bifida.

neuritis inflammation of a nerve.

neuroblast embryonic nerve cell.

neuroblastoma a malignant (cancerous) tumour that develops from nerve tissue. It occurs in infants and children.

neurohormonal describes a harmonic relationship that exists between sensory and endocrine pathways. Hormones from the endocrine system react and interact with the nervous system. Stimulation from the nervous system produces an effect, e.g. the 'let-down' reflex during lactation or contractions during labour.

neuromotor referring to the working of nerves and muscles.

neuromuscular the nerves and muscles work together to achieve a desired state.

neuromuscular harmony different muscles behave differently but their behaviour is synchronised by the nervous system

neuron, neurone a single nerve cell.

neurosis a condition characterised by emotional instability. The psychological mood swings dramatically with small provocation.

neurotic prone to severe anxiety which causes changes of behaviour.

neutral in chemistry, neither acid nor alkaline.

neutrophil a type of white blood cell or leucocyte.

Neville Barnes forceps two curved blades which are applied to grip either side of the fetal head during the latter part of the second stage of labour. Traction is then applied and delivery of the fetal head is achieved.

newborn the name given to the baby after complete expulsion from its mother.

newborn screening test (NBST) offered to all newborns for early signs of a number of treatable congenital metabolic disorders. These include phenylketonuria, congenital hypothyroidism, cystic fibrosis and galactosaemia.

niacin part of the vitamin B complex—an essential nutrient in the diet required for maintenance of healthy skin, the gastrointestinal tract and the nervous system and the manufacture of sex hormones.

nicotine the toxic substance found in tobacco and now known to damage health and embryonic development.

nidation the embedding of the fertilised ovum in the endometrium of the uterus.

nipple the pigmented area in the centre of the breast which may or may not protrude.

nipple shield a concave, nipple-shaped latex cap which is applied over the nipple to theoretically protect the tissue from trauma during sucking.

nitrogen a gaseous element required for the formation of all protein substances.

nitrous oxide a gas which, combined with O_2 in a $50:50$ mix, can be inhaled as a mild analgesic in labour.

nocturia passing urine during the night; waking up to urinate.

nocturnal referring to occurrences during the night.

node a small rounded mass which can be palpated.

non-absorbable surgical suture material used to repair a surgical wound such as a perineal tear or episiotomy, which would otherwise be dissolved or ingested by enzymes in the tissues.

non-accidental injury damage occurring to the body by deliberate intention of another person.

non-binary those who do not identify as either male or female; they may identify as both or neither.

non-infective mastitis inflammation of the breast caused by a blocked milk duct.

non-invasive procedure diagnosis or treatment given without the need to penetrate tissues of the body.

non-invasive perinatal testing (NIPT) maternal blood test using circulating cell-free fetal DNA to screen for the more common aneuploidies (trisomies 13, 18 and 21 and Turner's syndrome).

non-maleficence the principle of 'first doing no harm'.

non-shivering thermogenesis the natural method for enabling the newborn to maintain its body heat by increasing its metabolic rate and burning stored brown fat.

noradrenaline a catecholamine secreted by the adrenal medulla and the nerve endings of the sympathetic nervous system and which causes vasoconstriction and increases in heart rate, blood pressure and blood sugar levels. It is both a hormone and a neurotransmitter.

normotensive having normal blood pressure.

notifiable disease any of a number of conditions, the occurrence of which must be made known to the director of public health of the health authority because they can be easily transmitted to other members of the community.

notification a legal obligation to inform authority representatives.

notification of birth the registrar must be informed of the birth of a baby so that a birth certificate can be issued and population statistics can be compiled.

NTDs *see* neglected tropical diseases.

nucha the nape (lower posterior aspect) of the neck.

nuchal relating to the nape of the neck.

nuchal cord an umbilical cord that is wound around the neck of the fetus during birth.

nuchal displacement a complication of breech labour, when an arm is displaced behind the child's neck.

nuchal fold layer of skin and underlying fat over the back of the neck which can be scanned by ultrasound at an early stage of gestation to measure the thickness (*see* Fig. 68; *see* nuchal translucency). A thickened nuchal fold suggests that further tests should be

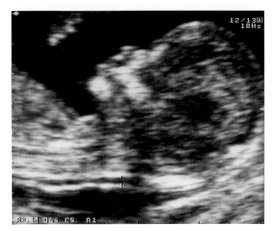

Figure 68
Nuchal fold scan

performed to investigate the possibility of the fetus having Down syndrome.

nuchal translucency an antenatal screening scan using ultrasound to help identify the chance of a woman having a baby with Down syndrome. The scan is carried out at 11–13 weeks' gestation and assesses the amount of fluid behind the neck of the baby.

nuchal translucency plus (NT Plus) maternal blood is taken about the time of the nuchal translucency ultrasound to increase accuracy of detecting babies at increased risk of chromosomal abnormality.

Blood testing includes PAPP-A (*see* pregnancy-associated plasma protein A) and B-hCG (beta-human chorionic gonadotrophin). All measurements combine to give a risk assessment for fetal chromosomal abnormalities.

nuclear family a small number of closely, usually biologically, related people living together.

nucleic acid one of a group of long chain proteins found in cells. There are two types: deoxyribonucleic acid (DNA) and ribonucleic acid (RNA).

nucleus the central structure in each cell which contains its genes and controls its behaviour.

nulliparous a woman who has not given birth to a live infant. WHO defines 'live' as showing any signs of life at the time of birth regardless of gestation.

numbness lack or loss of sensation or feeling.

nurture to feed, rear, foster, care for and enable the social development of children.

nutrition the process by which the body takes in and uses food to perform its functions, remain healthy and reproduce.

nymphomania a psychosexual disorder in women characterised by an insatiable desire for sexual intercourse.

nystagmus rhythmic, oscillating motions of the eyes.

O₂ a clear, colourless gas found in the atmosphere at 21% concentration. It is absorbed into the blood via the lungs and is essential for all bodily activities.

OA *see* occipitoanterior.

obese describes someone with a normal-sized skeleton but with a larger than normal amount of soft tissue, causing the body mass index (BMI) to be high.

obesity an excess of fat cells, mainly in the subcutaneous tissue.

objective 1. of a mind or minds, independent. 2. being evident to other people; measurable. 3. not influenced by personal feelings.

oblique at a slant, not horizontal or vertical.

oblique presentation where the long axis of the fetus (spine) is lying oblique or slanted in relation to the long axis of the uterus.

observation something which is seen or noticed.

obstetric forceps surgical instruments with handles attached to a blunt blade used to surround and apply traction to the fetal head in order to achieve birth.

obstetrician a doctor who has received additional education and experience in obstetrics and the management of pathological conditions which may occur in pregnancy, childbirth and the puerperium.

obstetrics the branch of medicine concerned with caring for women in pregnancy, childbirth and the puerperium.

obstipation intestinal obstruction; severe constipation.

obstructed labour an arrest or interruption to the process of giving birth due to a restriction in the birth canal.

obturator a device applied to block a space, canal or passage.

occipital referring to the region at the back of the head, just above the neck.

occipital bone the cup-like bone at the back of the skull marked by a large opening called the foramen magnum.

occipitoanterior (OA) relationship of the fetal head within the maternal pelvis. The back of the fetal head is to the front of the maternal pelvis.

occipitobregmatic diameter of the fetal skull taken from below the occipital protrusion to the anterior fontanelle. In the average term baby it is approximately 10.5 cm. When measured from below the occiput it is the suboccipitobregmatic diameter and is slightly shorter at 9.5 cm.

occipitofrontal diameter of the partially deflexed fetal skull measured from the occipital protrusion to the forehead. It is 11.5 cm in the average term fetus.

occipitolateral a position of the fetal head in relation to the maternal pelvis where the occipital bone is to the side of the mother's pelvis.

occipitoposterior (OP) a position of the fetal head in relation to the maternal pelvis where the occiput is to the back of the pelvis. This is not ideal for labour as the head will either have a long rotation in order to accommodate the curve of the birth canal or will descend through the birth canal in this position (persistent occipitoposterior position), possibly being born face-to-pubes.

occiput the bone at the back of the fetal head and in particular the central part which protrudes.

occlusive cap used as a method of contraception, it is introduced by the woman via the vagina and is applied so that it completely covers the cervix. Often used with a spermicide.

occult hidden, concealed.

oedema collection of fluid in the tissues of the body.

oesophageal referring to the oesophagus.

oesophageal atresia a congenital abnormality in which the oesophagus ends in a blind loop before reaching the stomach (*see* Fig. 69). It may be suspected in pregnancy by the presence of polyhydramnios and may be seen on ultrasound scan. It may be suspected in the neonate who only takes small amounts of its feed or vomits undigested milk. Surgical correction is required urgently.

oesophagus the muscular tube which passes food from the back of the throat into the stomach.

oestrogen, estradiol, estriol, estrone hormones from the ovary or placenta which have various effects on the body influencing growth of breast tissue and fat deposits at puberty, development of the lining of the uterus on a monthly cycle ready for implantation of a fertilised ovum, growth of the uterus and breasts in pregnancy, water and electrolyte retention and inhibition of lactation during pregnancy.

oestrogenic a substance (e.g. a plant, herb or pharmaceutical drug) whose effects resemble those of oestrogen.

oestrone *see* oestrogen, estrone.

olfactory referring to the sense of smell.

olfactory nerve the cranial nerve which passes directly

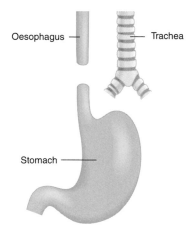

Oesophagus — — Trachea

Stomach —

Figure 69
Oesophageal atresia

from the brain to the nose or nasal area.

oligaemia reduction in the volume of blood.

oligo-, olig- combining form meaning deficiency of, few.

oligohydramnios deficiency in the volume of the amniotic liquor around the fetus in utero. This is associated with congenital abnormalities of the kidney and intrauterine growth restriction.

oligomenorrhoea a slight reduction in menstrual blood loss.

oligospermia a deficiency in the number of sperm in the semen. It is associated with subfertility.

oliguria a deficiency in the volume of urine secreted by the kidney. It is associated with shock and renal failure.

ombudsman an official who investigates complaints about the health services. She or he passes evidence to a panel for jurisdiction.

omentum layer of connective tissues which is part of the peritoneum and which holds the stomach alongside its adjacent organs.

omphalocele a swelling around the umbilicus due to weakness in the muscular sheath over the abdominal cavity.

omphalus the umbilical cord.

o.n. (LATIN *omni nocte*, every night) an instruction to give a treatment, usually medicine, at night.

onco- word element meaning tumour, swelling, mass.

one-to-one midwifery a model of maternity care provided by one midwife (with a back-up midwife) that focuses on providing midwifery continuity of carer through pregnancy, labour and birth, and early parenting.

ooblast a primitive cell in the ovary from which the ovum develops and emerges.

oocyte an ovum released but at an immature stage, so a conception is unlikely to be successful.

oophor-, oophoro- combining form meaning ovary.

oophorectomy surgical removal of the ovary.

oophoritis inflammation of the ovary.

oophorosalpingectomy surgical removal of the ovary and the fallopian tube.

OP *see* occipitoposterior.

operation surgical treatment.

operculum the thick plug of mucus found in the cervical canal during pregnancy. It prevents infection entering the uterus and forms the 'show' during the early stages of labour because it emerges as the cervix begins to efface and dilate in response to contractions (*see* Fig. 70).

ophthalmia neonatorum an infection in the eyes of a newborn infant with purulent discharge caused by organisms in the vagina entering the eyes as the infant is born. It may be very serious with consequences for the future sight of the infant.

ophthalmoscope an instrument with a light and a lens used for examining the eyes.

opiate a strong drug derived from opium. It causes sleep or relief from pain. Its use is controlled by statute as it is a drug of addiction (*see* controlled drug).

opinion the advice offered by an expert (a judicial court or a midwifery or medical consultant).

opioid a drug derived from the poppy plant (i.e. morphine) with opium-like effects on the body. Endorphins and enkephalins produced in the body are thought to be natural opioids.

opium a drug made from unripe capsules of poppies used to manufacture morphine and other very strong drugs.

opportunistic infection an infection which occurs only because the body's defences have been weakened by another recent or current pathological condition.

opsonin a substance which coats bacteria or other cells making it easier for leucocytes to work and destroy them.

optic relating or referring to the eye.

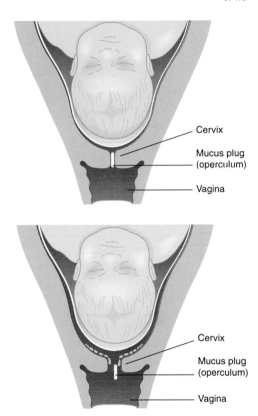

Cervix

Mucus plug
(operculum)

Vagina

Cervix

Mucus plug
(operculum)

Vagina

Figure 70
Operculum

optimal cord clamping (SYNONYM delayed cord clamping) waiting for umbilical cord pulsations to cease prior to clamping and cutting thus optimising the newborn's blood volume.

oral refers to the mouth.

oral contraceptive pill a tablet taken by mouth daily which aims to prevent a woman becoming pregnant.

orbit a circular structure, usually referring to the bony cavities in the skull which house and protect the eyeballs.

orbital ridge the upper bony aspect of the orbital cavity, which if felt on vaginal examination indicates a fetus presenting by the brow.

orchi-, orchido- combining form meaning the testes.

orchiopexy an operation in which an undescended testicle is loosened from restraining tissues and brought into the scrotum and attached so that it cannot be retracted.

orchitis inflammation of the testis.

organ a group of tissues in the body, usually encapsulated, which have a particular function.

organic a chemical compound containing carbon.

organism a living being, plant or animal.

organogenesis the process during early embryonic life by which the cells of the body migrate to the appropriate sites and become specialised to the function they must perform.

orgasm the climax of masturbation or the sexual act involving strong muscular contractions of the reproductive organs and accompanied in males by ejaculation of semen.

orifice an opening into or out of a cavity or organ.

oropharynx the part of the throat immediately behind the mouth and below the nose.

-orrhaphy suffix which refers to repair or suturing of something, as in *colporrhaphy*, surgical suturing and repair of the vaginal wall.

orthopaedics the branch of Western medicine concerned with bones and muscles.

orthostatic relating to or caused by standing upright, as hypertension.

Ortolani's test a test done on the hips of newborn infants to detect dislocation.

os 1. bone. 2. mouth or opening. The *cervical os* is the mouth or opening of the uterus. The *external os* is the part of the cervix which forms the opening into the vagina. The *internal os* is the part of the cervix which forms the opening into the uterus.

os innominatum (innominate bone) the three fused bones on either side of the pelvis which form the girdle.

Osiander's sign pulsation of the uterine arteries felt through the walls of the vagina, a sign said to be a presumptive indicator of pregnancy.

osmolality refers to the pressure of a fluid.

osmosis the movement of a pure solvent such as water across a permeable membrane from a solution that has a lower concentration to one of a higher concentration. The movement of fluid continues until the concentration is equal on both sides of the membrane.

osmotic pressure the pressure felt by a semipermeable membrane which divides a strong solution from a weaker one.

ossification the development of bone by the laying down of calcium.

osteomalacia a condition arising in normally formed bones whereby calcium is lost due to inadequate dietary intake of vitamin D or the minerals calcium and phosphorus. The bones become soft, weak and painful. The equivalent in infants and children is rickets.

osteomyelitis inflammation of bone, localised or generalised, due to infection, usually by pyogenic organisms.

osteopathy a form of treatment to correct imbalances in the musculoskeletal system. Diagnosis and correction is by manipulation and massage.

otitis infection of the ear.

-otomy suffix indicating cutting into.

outlet the route by which exit is achieved.

outlet contracture refers to the pelvis in the rare circumstance where the bones are too close together to allow the fetus to pass through.

output the total amount produced. *Cardiac output* is the amount of blood the ventricles pump out in a specific time (usually 1 minute).

outreach clinic a clinic away from a main hospital site which may be in a local centre where it is more accessible to the community or a specific group in the population.

ova *see* ovum.

ovarian referring to the ovary.

ovarian cyst a globular sac, filled with fluid or connective tissue, on the ovary.

ovarian follicle a small cavity on the ovary which contains a fluid dividing the follicular cells into layers and surrounds an ovum.

ovarian hyperstimulation syndrome (OHSS) a response to fertility treatment where women may develop severe fluid retention and abdominal swelling.

ovarian pregnancy a pregnancy which becomes implanted on the wall of or within the ovary. It does not usually survive.

ovariotomy cutting into the ovary. Usually refers to removal of the ovary.

ovary an almond-sized organ found in the broad ligament on either side of the uterus. The ovaries are responsible for producing and maturating an ovum each month and the secretion of the ovarian hormones oestrogen and progesterone. Ovarian activity is governed by the pituitary gland which secretes follicle-stimulating hormone (FSH) and luteinising hormone (LH). Oestrogen and progesterone form a negative feedback loop in which the pituitary produces less FSH in response to rising levels of oestrogen and less LH in response to rising levels of progesterone. The oestrogen and progesterone cause the lining of the uterus to become thickened and congested with blood in readiness for receipt of a fertilised ovum.

overdose an excessive concentration of a substance in the blood which will cause side effects and could result in altered consciousness, coma or death.

ovulation the expulsion of a mature ovum from the ovary, a process occurring on average 14 days before the period is due.

ovulation induction when fertility medications are used to stimulate growth and release of the eggs.

ovum (PLURAL ova) the reproductive cell produced by the female body on a regular basis which contains half the chromosomes required to form a conceptus.

oxygen an element found in the form of a gas essential to life. It is clear, colourless and found in a 21% concentration in the atmosphere. It is drawn into the lungs during respiration and crosses the membranes of the alveoli to combine with haemoglobin to form oxyhaemoglobin.

oxyhaemoglobin the substance found in the blood which is haemoglobin and oxygen combined. In this way oxygen can easily be transported around the body and released into cells with a low concentration.

oxytocic the name given to a substance which will cause contractions of the uterus.

oxytocin a hormone produced by the posterior pituitary gland which causes contraction of uterine muscle and the lactiferous tubules of the mammary glands, forcing milk towards the nipple. It can now be produced synthetically and is used to induce contractions in the first and second stage of labour and to control postpartum haemorrhage.

Pp

PO₂ partial pressure of oxygen.

P$_a$CO$_2$ the part of the total blood gas pressure exerted by carbon dioxide. Normal values are 35–45 mmHg in arterial blood and 40–45 mmHg in venous blood.

P$_a$O$_2$ the part of the total blood gas pressure exerted by oxygen. In arterial blood it should be 95–100 mmHg.

pachyonychia congenita a congenital ectodermal defect characterised by thickening of the nails, hard skin on the palms and soles, abnormality of the hair follicles and overgrowth and thickening of the skin of the knees and elbows.

pachyvaginitis an inflammation and thickening of the walls of the vagina.

packed cells blood cells which have been concentrated down into a smaller volume by centrifuging. Used to treat severe anaemia.

packed cell volume (PCV) refers to the amount of red cells in a litre of blood. The normal value is around 45%.

packing material inserted into a wound to ensure slow healing by granulation.

pad wad of soft material used to apply pressure on the body, act as a cushion or absorb moisture including menstrual blood.

paediatrics the branch of medicine concerned with health and disease in children.

paediatrician doctor who specialises in the care of children.

paedophilia condition of an adult with an abnormal interest in sex with children.

pain a sensation caused by stimulation of the sensory nerve endings. It is a subjective sensation with different individual responses and may be perceived as unpleasant and uncomfortable or as a positive bodily message. It is a cardinal symptom in the diagnosis of inflammation, trauma and neoplasm. Pain can be described as mild, dull, acute, generalised, burning, sharp, stabbing or referred. A person in pain may appear distracted, self-focused, narrow focused with altered time perception, to have altered thought processes, and to limit interaction with other people.

pain gate theory see gate control theory of pain (*also see* Fig. 71).

pain in labour this is caused by the uterus contracting and the cervix dilating and is a

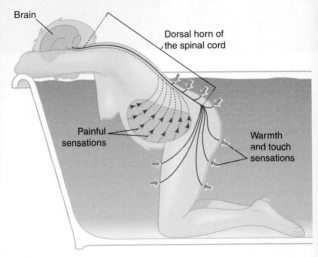

Figure 71
Pain gate theory

normal part of labour. The pain is characteristically intermittent, felt in the lower abdomen and sometimes the sacral region, and increases in frequency and intensity. The exact cause is unknown but theories have been advanced that it may be caused by one or a combination of the following features: stretching of the cervix; ischaemia as the uterine contractions reduce the blood flow; and/or pressure on the supporting ligaments.

pain receptor the nerve fibre endings which are found throughout the body. They are stimulated by pressure or heat and their impulses are interpreted by the brain as pain.

palate the roof of the mouth. It is hard at the front and soft at the back. It divides the nose from the mouth. Part of it may be absent due to developmental anomaly and the baby is born with a cleft palate.

pallid pale, skin without colour.

palmar crease the tiny grooves found running across the inside of the clenched hand.

palmar grasp reflex the ability of a newborn to strongly grasp an object which touches the palm of its hand.

palmature a congenital abnormality in which the fingers are webbed one to another.

palpation an examination technique which uses touch. In *abdominal palpation* the abdomen is examined to detect abnormalities, to determine growth of a baby and to assess the lie, presentation, position and engagement of a baby.

palpitation fast beating of the heart which can be detected by physical signs.

palsy an abnormality in which some degree of paralysis is present.

pancreas a large gland found in the upper posterior part of the abdomen which manufactures hormones and enzymes that aid digestion.

pandemic describes an epidemic which is found throughout the population, or worldwide.

pang a sudden or severe spasm of short duration which evokes physical or emotional discomfort.

panic sudden and severe emotional disturbance which results in physical symptoms.

panic attack episode of acute anxiety, apprehension or terror which can cause immobility or strange behaviour.

panting fast, shallow breathing. It may be encouraged by some midwives in the second stage of labour during contractions to slow down emergence of the fetal head through the vulva with the goal of preventing damage to the perineum.

Papanicolaou test (SYNONYM smear, Pap smear or Pap test) a screening test in which mucus and cells are scraped off the cervix and examined microscopically to detect cells which may be abnormal or cancerous.

papilla a small nipple-shaped projection found in different parts of the body.

papilloma a small swelling, non-cancerous, formed of epithelial cells and white in appearance.

papule small raised area on the skin.

papyraceous like paper. A *fetus papyraceous* is one of twin babies who has died early in pregnancy and has been flattened by the surviving baby to resemble a paper cut-out.

para- prefix meaning near.

parabiotic syndrome transfusion of blood from one twin to another because of vascular anastomosis in the placenta. One twin will be anaemic and one plethoric.

paracentesis a sterile process during which fluid is drawn out of a body cavity. A small incision is made in the skin and a trocar is inserted to allow drainage.

paracervical around the cervix or neck of the uterus.

paracervical block anaesthesia caused by the injection of anaesthetic into the area which contains the nerves. May be used during an instrumental delivery.

paracervix the connective tissue of the pelvic floor extending from the uterine cervix to the side walls of the pelvic cavity.

paradigm a particular world view; a pattern used as a model to represent another set of connections, usually of concepts.

paraesthesia a strange sensation described as pins and needles. Experienced as a result of nerve pressure as in carpal tunnel syndrome or following an epidural anaesthetic.

paraldehyde a very strong-smelling liquid used to sedate or cause sleep. Can be given by a number of routes and is excreted by the lungs.

paralysis loss of sensation and/or movement caused by anaesthesia, trauma, disease, pressure or poisoning.

paralytic ileus loss of sensation and movement in the intestines, usually temporary and due to surgery or other severe illness. The abdomen is swollen and tender and bowel sounds are absent.

paramedic a person who has training in emergency medical care; some members of the ambulance service.

parameters a set of values within which normal and abnormal are defined. May also refer to boundaries, borders or limits of normality.

parametritis inflammation of the structures around the uterus.

parametrium the part of the connective tissue covering the uterus which extends sideways to cover the fallopian tubes.

paranoia a condition of the mind in which a person is suspicious of the people around them, who feels that other people are conspiring to harm them in some way, or has delusions or feelings of inferiority or greatness in one aspect of their life.

paranoid subject to feelings of paranoia.

paraphimosis retraction and constriction of the foreskin behind the glans penis making pulling it forward again difficult or impossible.

parasalpingitis inflammation around the fallopian tubes, usually due to infection.

parasite a smaller organism which lives on and relies for its survival on a larger one.

parasympathetic nervous system part of the autonomic nervous system. The parasympathetic nerves: slow the heart; stimulate peristalsis; cause tears, bile, insulin, saliva and digestive juices to be produced; dilate peripheral blood vessels;

constrict the pupils, oesophagus and bronchioles; and cause vasodilatation of the pelvic region allowing congestion of erectile tissue in both sexes.

parathyroid gland four small glands attached to the upper poles of the thyroid gland. They produce parathyroid hormone which helps maintain blood calcium levels, blood clotting, nerve reactivity and cell membrane permeability.

parenchymatous salpingitis inflammation of the functional layer of the fallopian/uterine tube.

parenteral the giving of drugs or treatment by a route other than the alimentary tract.

parenthood the state whereby an adult becomes responsible for the care and upbringing of a child.

paresis loss of function of motor nerve impulses to muscles but no loss of sensory nerve function.

parietal referring to the top of the head.

parietal bone two of the bones which cover the cranium and pass in a wide band across the top of the head with the anterior fontanelle at the front and the posterior fontanelle at the back.

parity number of previous pregnancies that a woman has had that have ended in a live birth or stillbirth.

parous having borne one or more live children beyond the 20th week of gestation.

paroxysm a sudden increase in the severity of symptoms, fit, seizure, convulsion or spasm.

partial placenta praevia the margin of the placenta is situated over the internal os of the cervix. When the os starts to dilate, that part of the placenta may separate causing potentially life-threatening bleeding to the mother and hypoxia to the fetus.

partial pressure the amount of pressure that can be exerted by one gas in a mixture of gases or a liquid. The amount of pressure is dependent on the concentration of that gas in the mixture.

partnership in midwifery practice, partnership means working with the woman in a relationship of trust, shared decision-making and responsibility, negotiation and shared understanding.

partogram a graphic record of the progress of labour, particularly the dilation of the cervix and descent of the head seen alongside observations of the wellbeing of the mother and fetus.

parturient relating to the process of giving birth to a baby.

parturition the process of giving birth.

pascal (Pa) an international unit by which pressure may be measured.

passive doing nothing; not active.

passive immunity protection from a disease or infection

acquired by a person without action or reaction being required on their part. A fetus obtains this from its mother via the placenta and a neonate via the breast milk.

pasteurisation the process of heating milk to 60°C for 30 minutes so that some of the most harmful bacteria (e.g. tuberculosis) will be killed.

pasteurised milk milk which has been treated by pasteurisation.

Patau's syndrome congenital abnormality of the chromosomes (trisomy 13), where the infant has misshapen hands, face and feet and mental disability.

patent open.

patent ductus arteriosus an abnormal condition in which there is a persistence of the fetal circulation, an opening between the aorta and pulmonary artery enabling the larger volume of blood to bypass the lung with reduced oxygen uptake (*see* Fig. 72).

paternity refers to the state of having fathered a child.

paternity suit when a mother applies to the courts for money from a man she claims to be the father of her child. In some cases paternity is proved or disproved by DNA testing.

patho-, path-, -pathy combining forms meaning disease.

pathogen an organism which causes disease or infection.

pathologist a person specially trained in the study, detection and tracking of pathogens.

pathology 1. a branch of science which deals with the nature, cause and progression of disease. 2. the study of disease-causing organisms, usually in a laboratory.

patient person receiving healthcare; generally used to refer to people who are sick rather than healthy childbearing women.

patient-controlled analgesia (PCA) self-regulation of analgesia. Usually reserved for use after major surgery. The analgesia (usually narcotic) is prepared and connected to an IV site and syringe pump and the patient depresses a plunger to deliver it. A safety lock-out system prevents overuse/overdose.

patulous referring to something that is open or spread apart. May refer to the cervical os in the postnatal period.

Pawlik's grip a method of assessing engagement of the presenting part during pregnancy. The index finger and thumb of one hand are applied just above the symphysis pubis and the presenting part is ballotted. It can be painful for the mother and is not recommended in practice.

PCO₂ the pressure of carbon dioxide in the blood. Normally it is 40 mmHg.

PCR *see* polymerase chain reaction.

PCV (packed cell volume) refers to the amount of red blood cells in a litre of blood.

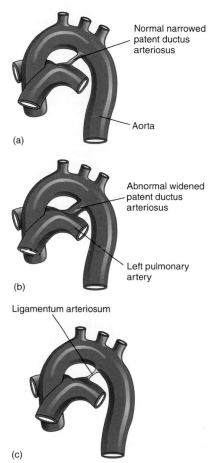

Figure 72
Patent ductus arteriosus

pectineal of or relating to the pubic bone.

pectoral referring to the breast or chest, or the large muscles over the breast and thorax: pectoralis major and minor.

pedigree line of descent through the generations of a family. Some diseases can be traced from one generation to another.

peduncle a large stalk or pedicle.

peak inspiratory pressure (PIP) a measurement used to assess the highest level of pressure in the lungs during inhalation.

PEEP *see* positive-end expiratory pressure.

peer review a means of evaluating the professional practice of a colleague of equal status according to preset standards, and done as part of an audit of the service.

pellagra a deficiency of niacin and protein in the diet can lead to this disease. The effects include skin eruptions, digestive and nervous system disturbances and eventual mental deterioration.

pelvic referring to the pelvis.

pelvic bones the innominate bones (fusion of the ilium, ischium and pubis) which form the pelvic girdle along with the sacrum and symphysis pubis.

pelvic brim the part of the pelvis which the baby enters before or during labour. The brim is bordered by the symphysis pubis, superior ascending ramus, sacroiliac joints, iliopectineal lines, ala and sacral promontory.

pelvic congestion increase in blood volume supplying the organs in the pelvis; found in early pregnancy and just before a woman's period is due.

pelvic examination an examination performed by inserting two fingers into the vagina to feel the size and shape of the pelvis, and the position and condition of the organs.

pelvic floor the two layers of muscles lying across the outlet of the pelvic girdle.

pelvic floor exercises exercises done to tighten and tone the muscles of the pelvic floor.

pelvic haematoma extravascular collection of blood; if sufficiently large it may cause pain and pressure sensations.

pelvic inflammatory disease (PID) severe illness originating from infection of the genital tract which has spread to the pelvic reproductive organs. Can lead to infertility.

pelvic inlet the first area of the bony pelvis through which a fetus will pass during birth (*see* Fig. 73).

pelvic outlet the last area of the pelvis through which the fetus will pass during birth (*see* Fig. 73).

pelvimetry measuring the diameters of the pelvis.

pelvis the bony girdle formed by the pelvic bones and closed at the lower aspect by

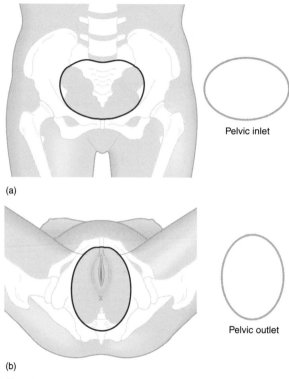

(a)

Pelvic inlet

(b)

Pelvic outlet

Figure 73
Pelvic inlet and pelvic outlet

the pelvic floor muscles (*see* Fig. 74). The organs contained within the girdle are the bowel, rectum, bladder, uterus, fallopian tubes and ovaries.

pemphigus a group of immune-mediated diseases of

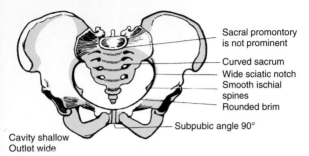

Sacral promontory is not prominent

Curved sacrum
Wide sciatic notch
Smooth ischial spines
Rounded brim

Subpubic angle 90°

Cavity shallow
Outlet wide

Figure 74
Pelvis

the skin and mucous membranes characterised by vesicles, bullae, erosions and ulcerations.

pendulous hanging down loosely, dangling.

pendulous abdomen the pregnant abdomen hangs down when the abdominal wall muscles are weakened by a large number of previous pregnancies or large babies.

penetrate to enter, maybe with difficulty.

penis male organ made of erectile tissue and through which passes the urethra for the transport of urine and spermatozoa.

peptic referring to the stomach or digestive enzymes.

peptide a chain of molecules made up of amino acids (digested proteins).

per by, around, near to, enclosing.

per vaginam through the vagina.

percentile a term used in statistics. One percentile is a 100th part of the whole. The 80th centile means that 80% of the population being studied fall below a known or specified range and 20% above. *Percentile charts* are used to show the likely birth weight of babies at different gestations.

percussion tapping a part of the body and listening for vibrations to diagnose boundaries, size or contents of a body cavity.

perforate to make a hole in, or pierce.

performance indicators a means of measuring quality of care by a professional. May be done as part of a process of clinical auditing.

peri- prefix meaning around about an organ (e.g.

perimetric, relating to the *perimetrium*) or time period (e.g. *perinatal*, around the time of birth; *perimenopausal*, around the time of menopause).

pericardium the sac that encloses the heart and the roots of the great vessels. There are two layers: the visceral layer or epicardium, that surrounds the heart; and the outer parietal layer, which forms the sac and is lined with a serous membrane.

pericranium the membrane of connective tissue which surrounds or lines the inside of the skull bones.

periodontal disease advanced gum disease that may occur if gingivitis (early gum disease) is not treated. Periodontitis is linked with adverse perinatal outcomes including preterm birth.

perimetrium the membranes around the outside of the uterus.

perinatal around the time or process of birth.

perinatal death a fetal or neonatal death of at least 20 weeks' gestation or at least 400 g birthweight.

perinatal mortality the statistical expression of combined deaths per 1000 live births.

perineal refers to the perineum. Because of its position the perineum is vulnerable to trauma and infection during childbirth and it may need repair.

perineal trauma injury to the labia, anterior vagina, urethra or clitoris as a result of childbirth. Trauma may occur spontaneously during vaginal birth or by a surgical incision (episiotomy). Trauma is defined in the table in Appendix 4.

perineorrhaphy a surgical procedure in which the perineum is cleaned and repaired.

perineum the area of skin and muscle between the anus and the vagina which supports the internal organs of the pelvic cavity (*see* Fig. 75) and stretches to allow the baby to be born.

period an interval of time. In everyday language the term is used to describe the menses or menstrual period, the monthly loss of blood from the uterus as part of the menstrual cycle.

periodic apnoea of the newborn irregular pattern of breathing with rapid respiration followed by a period of apnoea present in the normal full-term infant.

periosteum the surface of a bone is covered by this thick fibrous membrane. It acts as an attachment for muscles and tendons.

peripheral at the extremities or ends, usually meaning the limbs.

peripheral resistance the failure of the blood vessels furthest from the heart to yield to its contractile forces.

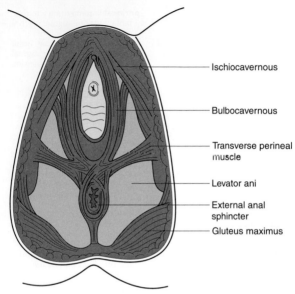

Ischiocavernous

Bulbocavernous

Transverse perineal muscle

Levator ani

External anal sphincter

Gluteus maximus

Figure 75
Perineum and supporting muscles

periphery the parts on the boundaries.

peristalsis the rhythmic muscular contractions which pass along a tube causing material in the tube to be pushed through.

peritoneum two sheets of membranes, the parietal peritoneum and the visceral peritoneum, the first of which lines the internal abdomen and the second the intestines.

The two sheets glide over each other and are lubricated by a little serous fluid.

peritonitis inflammation of the sheets of membrane (peritoneum) lining the abdominal cavity.

periventricular haemorrhage a bleed occurring into the cavities or around the ventricles within the brain. It occurs in preterm babies and can cause death. It is also an assumed cause of cerebral palsy.

permeable a membrane or sheet of tissue through which fluids can pass.

pernicious very harmful or destructive.

pernicious anaemia an anaemia due to the failure of the gastric juices to produce an intrinsic factor which allows absorption of vitamin B_{12}.

perodactyly congenital deformity of the fingers or toes including absence of some digits.

peropus congenital deformity of the feet.

persistent mentoposterior position this describes the position of the baby in the uterus where the head is fully extended and the face is presenting as the part likely to be birthed first. The chin is the denominator and is in the posterior quadrant of the pelvis. It does not rotate during labour. Vaginal birth is not always possible.

persistent occipitoposterior position describes the position of the baby in the uterus where the occiput is the denominator and lies closest to the mother's sacrum and even with good contractions does not rotate anteriorly.

personal protective equipment (PPE) any clothing or equipment used or worn to minimise risk to workers' health and safety.

person-centred care a framework that promotes respectful and responsive care provision based on the preferences, needs and values of the individual person.

perspire to sweat.

pertussis (SYNONYM whooping cough) a serious respiratory infection of bacterial origin for which a vaccination is readily available.

pessary a vaginal insert which can be a mechanical device used to maintain the uterus in an anteverted position or a large tablet-shaped object containing a drug which will be slowly released and absorbed through the vaginal mucus.

petechiae small red spots on the skin. Present on the face after delivery when the baby has had venous congestion. If it is present over the entire body it may suggest infection with rubella, cytomegalovirus or toxoplasmosis.

petit mal a mild form of epileptic fit. The person becomes unaware and unresponsive to their surroundings for a short period of time, as opposed to a grand mal attack which is a severe form of epileptic fit.

petroleum jelly a byproduct of refining crude oil. Used as a barrier or lubricating agent.

Pfannenstiel incision a surgical cut made across the lower abdomen just above the symphysis pubis. The most frequently used skin incision in caesarean section operations.

PG prostaglandin.

PGI₂ (prostacyclin), PGE₂ (dinoprostone) hormonally based gel or pessary inserted into the posterior fornix of the vagina to stimulate contractions of the uterus.

pH a tool of measurement used to express the concentration of hydrogen ions in a fluid, also referred to as the acid–alkaline balance. On a 14-point scale, 1 is strongly acid, 7 is neutral and 14 is strongly alkaline. Enzymes, gases and metabolic activity are enhanced by certain acid–alkaline media.

phagocytosis the process by which phagocytes will engulf and kill bacteria or other foreign materials.

phallic referring to the penis or an erect, penis-like shape.

phantom an image or impression; a device for stimulating the interaction of certain tissues with radiation.

phantom pregnancy the impression of being pregnant without evidence.

pharmacokinetics the study of drugs and how they behave in the body and with each other.

pharmacy a place for preparing and dispensing drugs.

pharynx the throat—a tube which extends from the base of the skull past the back of the mouth into the oesophagus. It allows the passage of air and food and can change shape during speech.

phenomenology a means of research by which the whole experience is studied. It focuses on describing experiences in order to deepen understanding of them.

phenotype an observable characteristic of an organism which may be physiological, biochemical or behavioural as a result of a combination of inherited traits and environmental factors.

phenylalanine an essential amino acid required for growth and development in infants. It is converted to tyrosine by an enzyme from the liver.

phenylketonuria (PKU) a congenital metabolic disorder characterised by the presence of phenylketones in the urine resulting from the incomplete conversion of phenylalanine to tyrosine. The blood levels will also be elevated; it can lead to permanent mental disability.

phimosis tight foreskin which cannot be drawn back over the glans penis. Hygiene is difficult, so infections can occur.

phimosis vaginalis a congenital condition in which the vagina is narrow or closed.

phlebitis inflammation of a vein, usually superficial but may be a deep vein in which case there is a risk of thrombosis (a clot) developing.

phlebothrombosis a clot of blood within a vein. It is usually in the calf muscle. There is a high risk of the clot becoming detached, travelling in the circulation to the lungs and becoming a pulmonary embolism.

phlebotomist a person who is trained to take blood from a vein.

phlebotomy the process of taking blood from a person.

phlegmasia alba dolens
inflammation which causes a
white leg as a result of a clot
in the femoral vein.

phobia fear or dread which can
be so strong that it disables
daily functioning. The person
may need counselling,
behavioural therapy or
psychiatric help.

phocomelia a baby born with
gross abnormality in
development of the long
bones. Hands, fingers, feet
and toes may be present.

phosphorus a chemical
element found in nature. It is
essential in the body for
using protein, calcium and
glucose.

photophobia an intense dislike
of light, a symptom of
meningitis.

photosensitivity an excessive
response of the skin to
sunlight or ultraviolet
radiation that may be caused
by certain disorders or
chemicals.

phototherapy treatment using
light rays. This accelerates the
breakdown of unconjugated
bilirubin so that the kidney
can excrete it. Bilirubin is a
byproduct resulting from
breakdown of fetal
haemoglobin which, until
removed from the circulation,
binds to fat and colours the
skin and sclera of the eye
yellow. It is commonly
referred to as jaundice.

phrenic of or relating to the
mind or the diaphragm.

physiological breech birth the
spontaneous birth of a baby

presenting by the breech
without interference, medical
intervention or attempt at
extraction unless a problem
occurs.

physiological jaundice yellow
skin discolouration occurring
in 60% of neonates as excess
red blood cells are broken
down and the liver is not
quite mature enough to
conjugate them so they can
be excreted through the
kidneys.

physiological third stage
spontaneous expulsion of the
placenta and membranes
without intervention.

physiology the study of how
the body works.

pia mater the innermost
of the three meninges
covering the brain and
spinal cord.

pica a craving to eat substances
not normally considered fit
for food, e.g. clay, chalk.

PID see pelvic inflammatory
disease.

pie chart a means of
representing numerical
information on paper in
the form of a circle so that
percentages of the whole
are easily visualised.

Pierre Robin syndrome
congenital abnormalities
including a small mandible,
cleft lip and palate, and other
defects of the eyes and ears.
Intelligence quotient is
usually normal.

pigment colouring of the
skin and hair resulting
from the presence of
melanin.

piles (haemorrhoids) varicosities protruding from the anus.

pilonidal of or relating to a growth of hair in a dermoid cyst or in the deeper layers of the skin.

Pinard's stethoscope a trumpet-shaped instrument used for listening to the fetal heart sounds through the abdominal wall.

pineal body a cone-shaped structure in the brain whose function is unknown but is thought to be related to sexual arousal.

pinhole pupil very small pupil which may be congenital or the result of drugs.

pinna the projecting part of the external visible part of the ear outside the head; auricle.

pitting oedema small depressions left when fingers are pressed into tissues swollen by the presence of increased intercellular fluid.

pituitary gland pea-sized gland situated at the base of the forebrain behind the bridge of the nose. It secretes hormones which control the other endocrine organs.

PKU see phenylketonuria.

placebo a substance given to a person which has of itself no therapeutic properties but which may relieve symptoms because the person has been told that it will.

placenta the organ that feeds the baby during pregnancy. After birth of the baby the placenta is squeezed and separates from the wall of the uterus. In *abruptio placentae* the placenta starts to separate partially or completely during pregnancy, thereby reducing the blood supply to the baby who may die. In *battledore placenta* the cord is attached to the edge rather than centrally located. In *succenturiate placenta* the placenta has an additional lobe situated next to or near the main placenta (*see* Fig. 76). The succenturiate lobe may be detached from the main placental tissue and be retained during the third stage of labour, increasing the risk of haemorrhage and infection.

placenta accreta abnormal implantation of the placenta; occurs when the placenta has partially grown into the muscle of the uterine wall (myometrium) with partial or complete absence of the decidua basalis.

placenta bipartita a placenta which appears to have two halves or lobes.

placenta circumvallata a placenta which has a dense white ring on the internal surface caused by a double fold of chorium.

placenta increta abnormal implantation of the placenta; occurs when the placenta extends into the muscle of the uterine wall (myometrium).

placenta percreta when the placenta penetrates the entire uterine wall. This variant can lead to the placenta attaching

Blood vessels running through
the chorion from the placenta to
the succenturiate (accessory) lobe

Chorion

Umbilical
cord

Succenturiate
(accessory) lobe

Placenta

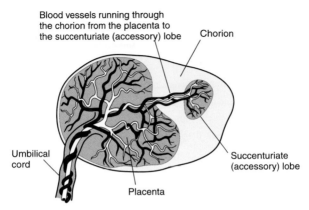

Figure 76
Placenta—succenturiate placenta

to other organs such as the
bladder.

placenta praevia describes a
placenta which implants in
the lower uterine segment. Its
margins may encroach on the
cervical os or the placenta
may entirely overlie the os.
Four grades are used to
describe the position of the
placenta: grade 1—the edge
of the placenta encroaches
into the lower uterine
segment; grade 2—the entire
placenta is in the lower
segment; grade 3—the
placenta reaches the internal
cervical os; grade 4—the
placenta covers the entire
cervical os. The placenta may
separate early in labour as the
os starts to dilate causing

bleeding and thereby
reducing the blood supply to
the baby causing compromise
or death.

placental barrier refers to the
membranes of the placenta;
they permit some substances
to enter while excluding
others.

placental encapsulation a
process of creating the
placenta into pills that can be
consumed, usually by the
mother. The process involves
steaming, dehydrating,
grinding and placing the
placenta into pills.

placental infarct death of an
area of the placenta. If this is
extensive it will reduce the
supply of nutrients and result
in fetal compromise including

intrauterine growth restriction.

placental insufficiency inability of the placenta to meet fetal demands. Development is compromised in severe cases.

placental lactogen a hormone similar to growth hormone which causes growth and development of the breasts during pregnancy.

placental membranes the amnion and the chorion which line the uterine cavity.

placental separation the means by which the placenta becomes detached from the uterine wall following the birth of a baby (*see* Fig. 77).

placentography radiological means of examining the placenta after injecting it with dye.

placentophagy refers to the eating of the placenta to ingest the hormones. It is believed to elevate the blood levels of oestrogen and progesterone and possibly prevent postnatal depression.

plagiocephaly an asymmetric condition of the head, due to irregular closure of the cranial sutures.

plantar refers to the sole of the foot.

plasma straw-coloured part of the blood made up of water, electrolytes, gases, proteins, glucose, fats and bilirubin. In it are suspended blood cells, erythrocytes, leucocytes and platelets.

plasma expander fluids of high molecular weight given intravenously to raise the blood pressure in situations of shock or haemorrhage.

plasma protein the collective name given to albumin, fibrinogen, prothrombin and gamma globulins, substances which maintain water balance and blood pressure and create osmotic pressure.

plasma volume the amount of plasma in the body. It will be reduced by shock, haemorrhage and dehydration.

plasmin an enzyme which dissolves the fibrin in a thrombus (clot).

platelets (thrombocytes) cells in the blood which are disc-shaped and are essential to coagulation. They stick to uneven or damaged surfaces causing occlusion through the formation of a clot.

platypelloid word used to describe a pelvis with wide lateral diameters and reduced anterior–posterior diameters. Women with platypelloid pelves rarely have difficulty in labour but the fetal head is unlikely to engage before labour.

plethora excess, usually of red blood cells.

plethoric having the appearance of being saturated with blood.

pleura two membranes, one surrounding the lungs and the other the thorax. The membranes are in very close proximity to each other with only a little fluid between to lubricate them.

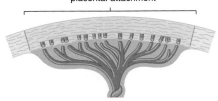

Area of
placental attachment

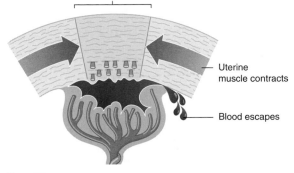

Area of
placental separation

Uterine
muscle contracts

Blood escapes

Figure 77
Placental separation

pleural cavity the space in the thorax occupied by the lungs and heart.

plexus a place where a number of nerves meet. The *brachial plexus* is the network of nerves which supply the arm.

plurality the number of births resulting from a pregnancy.

pneumococcal meningitis serious infection of the meningeal membranes by *pneumococci* bacteria.

pneumococcus common term for the bacterial infection-causing organism *Diplococcus pneumoniae*.

pneumonia inflammation of the lung due to infection. May affect all or part of the tissue.

pneumonitis inflammation of the lung, not necessarily due to infection but may be triggered by allergy or pollutants.

pneumothorax air or gas in the pleural space, resulting in collapse of the lung, usually as a result of trauma or some pathological process.

podalic of or relating to the feet; usually refers to internal podalic version, where the fetus is turned to a longitudinal lie by grasping one or both feet. Rarely used except in turning a second twin.

poison any substance taken into the body which causes changes in function detrimental to the body's welfare.

polarity term used to describe the harmonious working of the dominant upper uterine segment and the passive lower segment. Uterine contractions in the fundus are strong, and lose strength as they travel towards the lower segment which relaxes and dilates with the cervix as the labour progresses (see Fig. 78).

pole either extremity of an axis, as of the baby, or of an organ of the body, e.g. the uterus.

poliomyelitis a viral infection of the spinal cord. It is transmitted by the oral–faecal route and may present as nothing more than a common cold. It can, however, cause large muscles of a limb to become paralysed or involve the muscles of respiration and the patient frequently dies. It is a notifiable disease. Live attenuated virus is used in preparation of oral vaccines offered to infants at 2, 3 and 4 months of age; the vaccine itself occasionally transmits the disease.

pollutant a substance in the air which when inhaled undermines the body's wellbeing.

poly- combining form meaning many or much.

polycystic many small cysts or swellings containing fluid or other material.

polycystic kidneys kidneys which are enlarged by many small cysts.

polycystic ovaries ovaries which contain many small cysts. They do not function normally and the woman may experience infertility.

polycystic ovarian syndrome (PCOS) disorder that is associated with polycystic ovaries and has a genetic element.

polycythaemia an excess of red blood cells. Newborn babies are usually polycythaemic, the haemoglobin being of the fetal type which is quickly broken down but not so quickly excreted, leading to physiological jaundice.

polydactyly having an extra digit on the hand or the foot.

polyglactin a substance that is found in absorbable sutures.

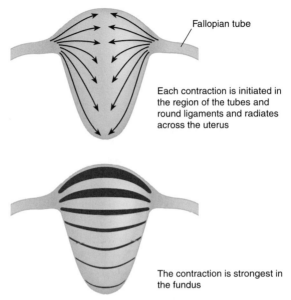

Fallopian tube

Each contraction is initiated in the region of the tubes and round ligaments and radiates across the uterus

The contraction is strongest in the fundus

Figure 78
Polarity

polyhydramnios having an excess of fluid in the uterine cavity during pregnancy (*see* Fig. 79). It may be suggestive of fetal abnormality (e.g. oesophageal atresia).

polymerise chain reaction (PCR) a laboratory testing process used to directly detect the presence of an antigen, rather than the presence of the body's immune response or antibodies.

polymorphic the ability to appear in two or more forms, such as the existence of two or more forms of chromosomes or haemoglobins in a population.

polyneuritis inflammation involving many nerves.

polypus (SYNONYM polyp) a small tumour on a stalk attached to a mucous membrane. May be found on the cervix, containing placental tissue, or resemble a small fibroid.

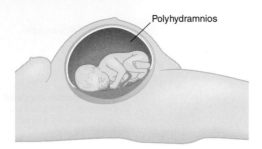

Figure 79
Polyhydramnios

---

polyuria passing a lot of urine.

pons that part of the brain lying between the medulla oblongata and the mid-brain.

popliteal space the space at the back of the knee joint.

pore a minute opening in tissue serving as an outlet for perspiration.

portal vein the large vein which carries nutritive material from the digestive tract to the liver.

port-wine stain (SYNONYM naevus flammeus) a patch of red/purple discolouration of the skin present at birth.

position usually refers to the attitude of the woman in labour, standing, squatting, forward-leaning, on hands and knees, lying prone, supine, recumbent, knee–chest (in cases of cord prolapse to prevent the cord being occluded), left lateral side, lithotomy or Trendelenburg.

position of the fetus (*see* Appendix 3 for diagrams) the relationship of the presenting part of the fetus to six points on the maternal pelvis. The presenting part, head or breech, has landmarks (denominator: occiput, mentum, sinciput, sacrum) used to describe the fetal aspect nearest to a given point on the pelvis. This landmark may be nearest to the anterior, lateral or posterior aspect of the pelvis on either the left or the right side. Commonly six positions are used: right occipitoanterior (ROA), right occipitolateral (ROL), right occipitoposterior (ROP), left occipitoposterior (LOP), left occipitolateral (LOL), and left occipitoanterior (LOA). If the denominator is the sacrum the same positions are used but sacro- (S) is used instead of occipito-. The same applies to the other denominators.

positive-end expiratory pressure (PEEP) the pressure remaining in the airways at the end of an inspiration–expiration cycle during mechanical ventilation. It is used to treat neonates with immature lungs. It keeps the alveoli and dead air spaces inflated and prevents collapse on expiration.

positive signs of pregnancy audible fetal heart sounds, fetal movements and visualisation of the fetus on ultrasound.

posseting regurgitation of a small amount of milk from the stomach of an infant after a feed.

post- combining form meaning after.

posterior fontanelle the soft fibromembranous point at the back of the infant's head above the occiput where three sutures meet (*see* Fig. 80). It may be used to define the baby's position on vaginal examination. It ossifies 6 weeks after birth.

posterior position the posterior fontanelle of the head lies nearest the mother's spine. The presenting diameter will not be optimal for labour. Backache, slow cervical dilation and descent of the head may be a feature of the labour as the head attempts to rotate to adapt to the shape of the pelvis.

postcoital contraception use of hormonal drugs after unprotected intercourse in an attempt to prevent fertilisation or implantation.

posterior at the back of.

posthumous after death.

postmature infant a neonate who displays features of dry peeling skin, long fingernails and toenails and skin folds that may crack.

postmenopausal vaginitis inflammation of the vagina associated with degenerative conditions due to hormonal reduction occurring after the cessation of periods.

postmortem (PM) (SYNONYM autopsy) examination after death to determine the cause of death.

postnatal after birth.

postnatal depression the negative mood and loss of motivation experienced by some mothers after childbirth. It starts between 10 days and 6 months after birth and can last up to 2 years.

postnatal period the time from birth up to 28 days during which the midwife should attend the mother and child.

postnatal psychosis a serious mental condition in which the woman is unaware of reality and can be a danger to herself or the baby. She may be admitted to a mother and baby psychiatric unit.

postoperative care the care provided after surgery until restoration of full consciousness and functioning state.

postpartum after labour.

postpartum haemorrhage (PPH) severe bleeding from the genital tract up to 6 weeks after labour, of 500 mL of blood or any

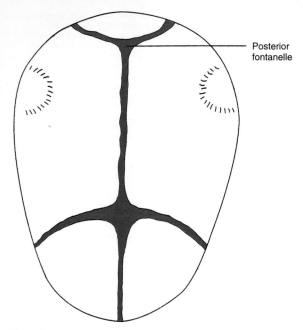

Posterior
fontanelle

Figure 80
Posterior fontanelle

amount which causes deterioration to the mother's health. May be a threat to the life of the mother requiring emergency management. Primary PPH occurs within 24 hours of birth and is due to relaxation of the myometrium. Secondary PPH occurs after the first 24 hours and up to 6 weeks postpartum and is due to infection or retained products of conception.

postprandial after a meal.

post-term describes a pregnancy which has lasted longer than the medically defined notion of 'term', usually considered to be between 37 and 42 weeks of pregnancy.

post-traumatic stress disorder a mental response caused by experiencing an acute emotional stress. It happens to people after a natural disaster and may occur in women who have experienced traumatic birth or abusive treatment during their childbirth experience.

postulate a theory; to theorise.

posture the position of the body and the limbs in relation to the trunk.

Potter's syndrome a set of features found in a baby without kidneys. They include poorly developed lungs, compression deformity and unusual facial characteristics. It is not compatible with life.

pouch a small pocket of tissue or membrane.

Poupart's ligament (SYNONYM inguinal ligament) found on the lower abdomen, it stretches from the superior ischial spines to the symphysis pubis.

poverty lacking in the resources and comforts which are expected as basic features of life.

PPE *see* personal protective equipment.

PPH *see* postpartum haemorrhage.

practitioner a person who has undergone a period of training and has satisfied the relevant professional regulatory body of their competence in the art and science required by that profession of its practitioners.

pragmatic a philosophy which believes that ideas are only valuable in terms of their consequences.

prandial pertaining to a meal.

preceptor a person who helps the learning of another without formal classes but by support and discussion.

preceptorship the system by which newly qualified practitioners are supported within the profession until they feel totally confident.

precipitate labour labour which is very fast, lasting less than 2 hours, and in which the contractions are intense.

preconception the time before embarking on a pregnancy and during which the woman is getting ready to conceive, possibly by adjusting her habits to a healthier way of life.

preconceptual care education and supportive advice provided by a healthcare worker or lay adviser to a woman or couples who are planning to become pregnant.

precursor something that precedes a condition or event.

pre-exposure prophylaxis (PrEP) a strategy whereby specific effective anti-HIV medications are offered as an additional prevention choice for pregnant women who are at substantial risk of HIV infection as part of combination prevention approaches.

pre-diabetes a condition where the blood glucose levels are higher than normal but not yet high enough to be diagnosed as diabetes.

predisposition a state of being susceptible or inclined to something.

pre-eclampsia (PE) the International Society for the Study of Hypertension in Pregnancy defines PE as the development of elevated blood pressure (systolic BP $\geq$ 140 mmHg and/or diastolic BP $\geq$ 90 mmHg phase 5) after the 20th week of pregnancy. Pre-eclampsia is usually first detected by the measurement of high blood pressure but features other than hypertension are required to make the diagnosis. Proteinuria is the most commonly recognised feature of pre-eclampsia after hypertension but pre-eclampsia affects other organ systems including the placenta (leading to fetal growth restriction).

pregnancy the state lasting 280 days during which the female nourishes in her body a fetus from conception until birth. An *ectopic pregnancy* is one where the conceptus is implanted in the fallopian tube or somewhere outside the uterus.

pregnancy test test done on blood or urine to detect a pregnancy. It is based on the detection of human chorionic gonadotrophin (hCG) produced by the trophoblast.

pregnancy-associated plasma protein A (PAPP-A) a protein produced by the placenta.

Although this test has poor sensitivity, a low PAPP-A is associated with increased adverse outcomes such as fetal growth restriction and preterm birth.

pregnanediol a progesterone-like substance found in the urine of pregnant women.

pre-implantation genetic testing (PGT) testing the genetic make-up of the embryo before it is transferred back into the woman.

premature early, the time before full development has been achieved.

premature infant an infant born before 37 completed weeks' gestation.

premature rupture of the membranes spontaneous rupture of membranes prior to term with the escape of amniotic fluid from around the fetus before the onset of labour.

premedication (premed) medicine, usually a sedative tranquilliser or hypnotic, given before an operation to reduce anxiety and prepare the body. Not usually given before a caesarean section because of the risk of side effects occurring in the fetus.

premenstrual the time 7–10 days before the start of the regular monthly bleeding which is part of the menstrual cycle.

premenstrual syndrome (PMS) uncomfortable symptoms of weight gain, breast tenderness, volatile mood swings and fatigue which may occur before menstruation.

prenatal before birth.

prenatal diagnosis test performed to confirm or exclude the possibility of a congenital abnormality following a positive screening test.

preoperative the time before an operation.

preoperative care routine procedures which are done before an operation to avoid the complications of anaesthetics; planning of the surgical procedure.

prepuberty the 2 years before menstruation during which secondary sex characteristics start to appear.

prepuce (SYNONYM foreskin) a loose fold of skin covering the end of the glans penis.

pre-registration midwifery education a midwifery training course for people wishing to become midwives. This may be 'direct entry' or after initial registration as a registered nurse.

prescription the order by which medicine is issued and given.

presentation the part of the baby which is lying in the lower segment of the uterus over the cervical os—can be cephalic (head) or breech.

presenting part the part of the baby which can be palpated in the lower pole of the uterus.

pressure force or stress which can be measured and compared to others.

pressure point the area over a bone where the arterial pulse may be felt. May be used for diagnosis and treatment in non-Western healing modalities. Specifically indicated points may be used in acupuncture or acupressure.

presumptive signs indications of a pregnancy, not necessarily beyond question, that is, amenorrhoea and morning sickness.

preterm before the full 37 weeks of gestation are completed.

preterm labour labour occurring before the 37th completed week of pregnancy. The baby is likely to be low birth weight.

prevalence the number of cases of a condition arising at a given time.

preventive measures to take measures so that a disease does not occur.

prevention of mother-to-child transmission (PMTCT) includes interventions to reduce the risk of HIV transmission from mother to baby including antiretroviral treatment for the mother and a short course of antiretroviral drugs for the baby as well as appropriate breastfeeding practices.

primary first or most important.

primary healthcare a way of providing healthcare which

recognises the importance of equity, access, affordability, the provision of services based on need, community participation, collaboration and community-based care.

primary healthcare teams small multidisciplinary groups of people who work from health centres and are often a person's first communication with midwifery or medical care.

primigravida a woman experiencing her first pregnancy.

primipara pregnant woman who has had no previous pregnancy resulting in a live birth or stillbirth.

primiparous having delivered one child.

primitive most basic, rudimentary, no evolution.

primitive groove the dent at the back of the embryonic disc which will become the cephalocaudal axis (head and spine).

primitive reflexes the behaviours with which the baby is born—sucking, breathing, crying, grasping, walking and Moro reflex.

privacy a cultural concept which allows a person to control the number of people around them and prevents intrusive behaviour by one person towards another.

private practice the work of a professional person who is not employed by an institution but is self-employed, may advertise services and make charges.

prn (LATIN *pro re nata*) an abbreviation used in prescriptions meaning give as needed.

probability a term used in reporting statistics which measures the likelihood of two or more parameters being related by more than chance.

problem-based learning (PBL) students are presented with a problem (trigger) and collectively discover what information they need to resolve the problem. They negotiate which member of their learning set will find which information and feed this back to the group on an agreed date.

procedure a sequential set of actions which together have a single purpose.

process 1. a series of events which will change one thing into another, one state will become another, or a condition will be resolved. 2. part of a bone.

procidentia the prolapse of an organ, usually the uterus which comes through the vagina.

procreation the process of conceiving, growing, birthing and nurturing children.

prodromal labour the early stage of labour when contractions occur but are not associated with progressive cervical dilatation.

prodrome the first symptoms which may lead to the diagnosis of a disease.

profession a large group of people with similar interests who have organised themselves, documented information and skills, regulated themselves (and by statute) and initiated novices after a course of training. They usually have skills which can be of service to the public and for which the public are willing to pay.

professional a person belonging to a profession who maintains the standards of service and practice adopted by that body.

professional liability the legal obligation of healthcare professionals to compensate their clients for acts of negligence in their professional practice which cause the clients suffering or damage. This is central to the concept of malpractice.

professional profile documented evidence of the professional person's practice and ongoing training or study.

profile a sketch, summary or diagram of a person or disease.

progeny offspring, children or descendants.

progesterone a hormone produced by the ovaries or placenta which is responsible for the thickening of the endometrium in the uterus, breast changes, water and electrolyte balance and the deposit of fat. It may be given as a medication to treat repeated abortions or for menstrual problems.

progesterone-only contraceptive a pill taken at the same time daily which aims to prevent the lining of the endometrium thickening to support implantation of a fertilised ovum. It can be taken by breastfeeding mothers as it does not inhibit milk secretion.

progestogen a natural or synthetic progestational hormone.

prognosis a prediction of the likely future or course of a disease or condition.

projectile vomiting strong spasm of the stomach muscles causing the contents to be ejected to a distance of many feet away from the patient. This symptom in a neonate indicates the presence of pyloric stenosis.

prolactin a hormone produced by the anterior lobe of the pituitary gland which is responsible for milk secretion.

prolapse falling of an organ from its usual position through a canal.

prolapse of rectum the protrusion of the rectal mucosal lining through the anus.

prolapse of the umbilical cord the umbilical cord falls through the cervical os in front of the presenting part and may become occluded by it if birth is not expedited or an emergency caesarean section is not performed.

proliferation highly productive, fast multiplication of cells.

proliferation phase refers to the second part of the menstrual cycle when the lining of the uterus is becoming thick and vascular.

prolonged labour slow cervical dilation taking more than 24 hours. Occasional risks to the mother include exhaustion, dehydration and ketosis. Risks to the fetus include hypoxia and abnormal moulding which may cause tears to the tentorium of the cerebellum and internal haemorrhage.

prolonged pregnancy pregnancy which lasts more than 42 weeks from the first day of the last normal menstrual period.

promontory that which sticks out. The *sacral promontory* is the part of the sacral vertebrae which protrudes into the pelvic cavity at the brim and reduces the anteroposterior diameter.

pronation of the hand the act of turning the palm posteriorly (or inferiorly when the forearm is flexed), performed by medial rotation of the forearm. May be used in manual rotation procedures to facilitate birth.

prone lying on the front aspect of the body, face downwards.

pronucleus the haploid nucleus of a sex cell.

prophylaxis a treatment given to prevent disease.

prostaglandin inhibitor an agent which prevents the production of prostaglandin and is usually a non-steroidal anti-inflammatory agent.

prostaglandins (PG) a group of substances first isolated in semen and which have an oxytocic effect, e.g. they cause increased smooth muscle tone and contractions.

prostate gland part of the male reproductive system located at the neck of the bladder which produces seminal fluid in which sperm may be transported and can swim.

prosthesis where a body part is replaced either internally (e.g. joint replacement) or externally (e.g. an artificial limb).

protein the part of the diet required for growth and repair of tissue. Contains the elements hydrogen, oxygen, nitrogen and carbon. It is digested in the stomach and absorbed in the form of amino acids, the most common being albumin (responsible for normal distribution of water throughout the body and the maintenance of the blood pressure).

proteinuria an abnormal condition where protein is excreted in the urine.

Proteus a bacterium normally found in the faeces but if transported to other parts of the body by contamination can cause urinary tract infections, pyelonephritis, wound infections and diarrhoea.

prothrombin a protein found in the plasma of the blood which in certain conditions will become thrombin in the presence of calcium and form part of a blood clot.

protocol a written plan which describes best treatment for a certain condition.

provider-initiated HIV testing and counselling (PITC) HIV testing and counselling which is routinely recommended by healthcare providers to persons attending healthcare facilities as a standard component of healthcare.

proximal next to, closest to.

pruritus itching sensation on the skin which causes a person to scratch.

pseudo- combining form meaning false.

pseudocyesis (false pregnancy) the woman feels she is pregnant and may develop symptoms of amenorrhoea and enlarged abdomen but there is no fetus in the uterus.

pseudohermaphroditism a name used to describe the fact that some people are born with external sex organs that look intermediate between the typical vagina or penis. Pseudohermaphroditism is not to be confused with hermaphroditism, in which the individual possesses both ovarian and testicular tissue.

pseudomenstruation bleeding which resembles a period but without changes in the lining of the uterus.

psych-, psycho- prefix meaning relating to the mind.

psychiatry a specialised branch of medicine which looks at disease processes of the mental, emotional or behavioural functions of the individual.

psychologist a professional who studies the structure of the brain and the functions of the mind.

psychomotor relating to motor activities, movements initiated at will.

psychomotor development the ongoing changes and refinement in mental and muscular harmony or cooperation. Usually refers to the progressive muscular control acquired at different ages.

psychoprophylactic preparation for childbirth education of parents concerning the processes of birth and how to cope with/ remain in control of them.

psychoprophylaxis a system for coping with pain in labour based on education in the Lamaze method of relaxation.

psychosexual relating to the mental and emotional aspects of sexuality.

psychosis severe mental illness characterised by delusions, hallucinations and illusions and loss of contact with reality. Postpartum, some women develop puerperal or postnatal psychosis.

psychosocial development progressive changes in a child's ability to interact with other people and develop relationships of trust and respect.

psychosomatic relates to the mind–body relationship where conditions felt psychologically may not have a physical basis.

ptosis the term used for a drooping upper eyelid.

ptyalin the enzyme in saliva which starts the process of starch digestion in the mouth.

puberty the transition in physical, mental and emotional functioning of the body which happens between about 10 and 18 years of age. The child emerges into adulthood.

pubescent uterus the body and cervix of the uterus are the same size and length in the adult as in the child.

pubic region the lowest part of the abdomen between the right and left inguinal regions.

pubic symphysis (SYNONYM symphysis pubis) the cartilaginous structure in the anterior midline of the pelvis. It may soften in pregnancy and the bones part causing symphysis pubis dysfunction.

pubiotomy the opening of the pubic bone in order to increase the pelvic diameters to let the baby pass through the birth canal.

pubis the bone at the front of the pelvis.

public health intervention in the environment and clinical practice which will affect the health of the population or community.

pubococcygeus that part of the pelvic floor muscle (levator ani) which stretches from the pubis to the coccyx.

pudendal refers to the external genital organs.

pudendal block anaesthetic injected into the region of the pudendal nerve before the application of forceps to anaesthetise the lower genital tract.

pudendum the external genitalia.

puerperal referring to the period of time after childbirth.

puerperal fever elevation of the temperature and other signs of severe infection following childbirth.

puerperal psychosis a severe mental illness which can follow childbirth.

puerperal pyrexia a rise in body temperature after childbirth.

puerperal sepsis infection, usually in the genital tract, after childbirth.

puerperium the period of time lasting 6–8 weeks after childbirth during which the body begins to return to its non-pregnant state and breastfeeding is established.

pulmonary referring to the lungs.

pulmonary circulation the flow of blood through the lungs so that oxygen can be taken up and pumped to the rest of the body and carbon dioxide given off.

pulmonary embolism a clot of blood which has travelled from another part of the body (the legs) and has become wedged in the small capillaries of the lungs, preventing flow and oxygenation of blood. It is accompanied by chest pain, cyanosis and tachypnoea. It can be life-threatening.

pulmonary surfactant a chemical found in the lung which maintains elasticity and inhibits collapse of the alveoli thereby facilitating gaseous exchange.

pulsation a throbbing or beating of an artery as blood passes through; it is rhythmic and in time with the beating of the heart.

pulse the rhythmic wave felt in an artery as the heart contracts forcing blood along it.

pulse rate the number of times per minute the heart pumps; the speed of the cardiac cycle.

pump apparatus used to move fluids from one place to another.

puncture making a hole in something by piercing it with a sharp instrument. In a *lumbar puncture* a hole is made in the meninges in the lumbar region of the spine in order to obtain cerebrospinal fluid for diagnostic or therapeutic purposes.

PUO (pyrexia of unknown origin) a body temperature above normal in response to something unknown.

pupil the apparently black circular opening in the centre of the iris of the eye, through which light passes to the retina.

purgative a medicine which causes the bowels to be evacuated or emptied.

purpura haemorrhagica purple spots or patches appearing on the skin or mucous membrane caused by bleeding of small capillaries beneath.

pus an exudate of yellow/white thick fluid which contains leucocytes, dead bacteria and skin cells. Produced in response to the body's resistance to an infection.

pustule small round patches on the skin with yellow tops indicating that pus is contained within.

pv (per vaginam) refers to medicine administered or examinations conducted by passing through the vagina.

pyaemia pus in the blood, a byproduct of bacterial invasion.

pyelitis infection in the renal pelvis of the kidney.

pyelonephrosis any disease of the kidney.

pyloric stenosis narrowing of that part of the gut that allows nutrients out of the stomach into the intestines for further digestion. Projectile vomiting and weight loss are the diagnostic features.

pylorus the opening between the stomach and the duodenum.

pyo- combining form meaning pus.

pyocolpos accumulation of pus in the vagina.

pyogen organisms/bacteria which produce pus.

pyogenic pus-forming.

pyometra accumulation of pus in the uterus.

pyosalpinx pus in the fallopian tubes.

pyretic referring to the presence of a fever or abnormally raised body temperature.

pyrexia fever, elevation in body temperature above normal in order to resist infection.

pyridoxine a preparation of vitamin B_6 given to treat anaemia.

pyuria pus in the urine, indicating the presence of infection in the urinary tract. The urine is cloudy.

Qq

QRS complex a series of letters denoting the parts of a cardiac muscular contraction so they can be recorded and analysed on paper (*see* Fig. 81).

quadrant a quarter of a circle or a part of the body which can be divided by four; the abdomen or the buttock (*see* Fig. 82).

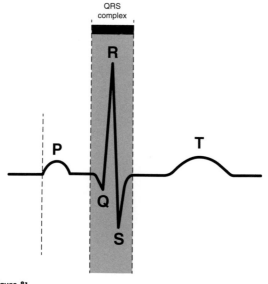

Figure 81
QRS complex
Illustration by Alan Laver

Quadrants

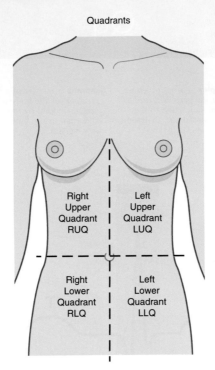

Figure 82
Quadrant
Illustration by Alan Laver

quadruplets four babies developing within the uterus or born in a single pregnancy.
qualified a person who has received recognised training and successfully completed the criteria for entering into employment requiring skills acquired during the training.
qualitative research a means of gathering and analysing information about life

experiences and their meaning. It is done to acquire information of a conceptual nature or about aspects of the human condition which vary from one individual to another.

quality assessment measures a system for evaluating patterns and programs of clinical, administrative and consumer care.

quality assurance a pledge or assurance given to the public by a group (service provider) that they will work towards certain standards of care which have been agreed by a multidisciplinary group.

quantitative research a means of research by which data are collected in numerical form; variables can be compared and interventions measured for effectiveness.

quarantine a period of time during which a person or animal thought to have been in contact with an infectious disease is isolated from contact with others. If after the expected time the person/ animal has not developed the infection, freedom to be in contact with others is restored.

quickening older term used for the moment in the pregnancy when the mother first feels the baby move. It happens around 19 weeks for a woman having her first baby and around 16 weeks for a woman who has given birth before.

quiet alertness the hour after a baby is born and several hours a day during which the newborn is calm and attentive, looks around and gets to know the adults around her/him and her/his environment.

quintuplets five babies developing within the uterus or born in a single pregnancy.

Rr

race a group of individuals with genetic and other characteristics in common.

racemose clustered; describes glands arranged around a central duct or orifice.

rachi-, rachio- prefix meaning of the spine.

rachischisis a congenital fusion of one or more vertebrae.

rachitic pelvis structural deformity of the pelvis caused by rickets in childhood.

radial referring to the radius bone in the lower arm.

radial artery the artery which passes down the arm and can be felt pulsating as it passes over the radius just above the wrist.

radial nerve large nerve supplying the arm and forearm.

radial nerve palsy damage to the nerve resulting in weakness and sensory loss which may be permanent or temporary following shoulder dystocia.

radiant describes an object which emits rays (of heat, light or electricity) or is the centre of rays which spread outwards.

radiate to diverge or spread out from a common point.

radiation the use of radioactive substances in diagnosis or treatment of disease.

radical dealing with the root or cause of a disease.

radical mastectomy surgical removal of the breast and extensive excision including lymph nodes, pectoral muscles and axillary lymph nodes to which cancerous cells may have spread.

radioactive a substance, usually metal, which emits electromagnetic vibrations.

radiographer a person trained to take and interpret X-rays of the bones and other parts of the body.

radiography examination by X-ray to detect or diagnose a condition. Not recommended in pregnancy without good clinical indications.

radioimmunoassay a means by which antibodies, antigens, hormones and drugs can be detected and measured.

radio-opaque something which stops the passage of X-rays and reflects them back so that an image can be created.

radiotelemetry a method of collecting information using a sensor and transmitting information to a base where it can be interpreted and recorded. Fetal heart monitoring can be recorded by this method.

radius one of the bones (with the ulna) in the forearm.

ramus the upper and lower arm-like parts of a bone as in the pubic bone.

random blood sugar or glucose test checking of blood sugar (glucose) level without prior preparation or warning. (*Compare* glucose tolerance test.)

random sampling a system in which research participants have an equal chance of being selected for a particular group.

randomisation the process by which individuals, e.g. experimental or control subjects, are allocated to groups, without a pattern or predictor of the group to which the subject will be assigned.

randomised controlled trial (RCT) a research method in which one group receives standard care and another group receives some form of intervention. Which participant is allocated to which group is decided completely by chance in an attempt to reduce bias.

rape sexual intercourse by force. The non-consenting party may be physically or psychologically injured by the assault. The term *medical rape* describes abuse arising from the application of medical procedures by force.

raphe a seam; line of union of the halves of various symmetrical parts.

rapport a sense of understanding, harmony and respect between two people.

rash raised red area of skin which can cause irritation. *Heat rash* appears in hot steamy conditions. It is also called prickly heat. *Nappy rash* appears over the nappy area and can be caused by irritation of strong urine (ammonia). It is more common where there is poor hygiene, and during colds, teething and earache.

raspberry leaf tea a herbal infusion often used in the latter part of pregnancy and thought to increase uterine muscle tone.

rate a measurement (e.g. of time, speed, velocity) used for the purpose of comparison. *Basal metabolic rate* is a unit of measurement used to indicate the body's requirements for oxygen when at rest. One person's rate can be compared with others and the result will be expressed in relationship to them. The *birth rate* is the number of births in a specific population over a period of time, usually expressed per year per 1000 of the population.

ratio a means of describing the quantity of one substance in relation to another. With the *lecithin–sphingomyelin ratio*, the relationship of these two substances to each other as found in the amniotic fluid is used to indicate fetal lung maturity.

rationale a system of reasoning or a statement of the reasons used in explaining actions or data.

Raynaud syndrome a condition in which arterial spasms in the fingers (and less commonly, the toes) cause reduced blood flow that usually lasts minutes but can last up to several hours. The episodes make the affected area become pale and then blue and there is often associated numbness or pain. As blood flow returns, the area turns red and burns. Can also affect nipples and may be a cause of nipple pain.

reaction a response occurring secondary to a treatment or stimulus.

reagent a substance which causes a reaction. It is a substance which in the presence of another to which it is sensitive alters its characteristics thereby indicating the presence of the other substance.

real-time scanner moving images created by ultrasound scanning.

reasonable care the degree of skill and knowledge expected of a qualified person.

recession drawing away from a normal position or turning backwards. *Sternal recession* is a sinking in of the breastbone with each inhalation seen in babies with respiratory distress syndrome.

recessive the opposite to dominant; a characteristic which will only be expressed as a genetic feature if a similar gene is present in both parents.

recipient the one who receives or accepts something given by another.

recommended daily allowance (RDA) the quantity of various nutrients in daily food intake recommended to be necessary for optimal health.

record permanent written communication which can be a document of care.

recovery return to normality or state of consciousness after an anaesthetic.

recreational drug a chemical substance not prescribed and taken for the pleasure it induces rather than for clinical indications.

rectal referring to the rectum, the lowest part of the alimentary canal closed by the anal sphincter. Drugs and infusions may be given and are well absorbed via this route.

rectal atresia the rectal canal ends in a blind loop and is not connected to the anal or distal end of the rectum (*see* Fig. 83).

rectal reflex the normal ejection response to the presence of an accumulation of faeces in the rectum. In babies this can be elicited within 20 minutes of a meal.

rectal temperature taken occasionally in the neonate; should be used with extreme caution as it carries risks of perforation. A special thermometer is required and the measurement is 0.4°C higher than the oral temperature.

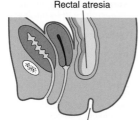

Rectal atresia

Anal canal

Proximal rectum

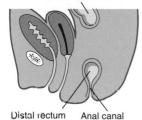

Distal rectum   Anal canal

Figure 83
Rectal atresia

---

rectocele a weakness in the muscle wall separating the rectum and vagina which allows the rectum and contents to bulge into the vagina. Surgical colporrhaphy may be performed to correct the defect.

rectovaginal refers to the rectum and vagina and the area where they are in closest proximity. In a rectovaginal fistula a hole appears between the rectum and vagina allowing faecal matter to leak out of the rectum into the vagina and out of the body in an uncontrolled manner.

rectovesical refers to the rectum and bladder.

rectum the lower 15 cm of the large intestine, it collects and contains faeces until it is convenient to evacuate.

rectus abdominis a pair of muscles on the anterior abdominal wall stretching from the ribs to the symphysis pubis. They may divide spontaneously during pregnancy and after delivery they can be palpated up to 4 cm apart. They usually close up within 6 months, especially with exercise, but occasionally surgical repair may be required.

recumbent lying down.

recurrent miscarriage defined as three or more miscarriages of a fetus before 20 weeks of gestation.

red blood cell count the number of erythrocytes in a specimen of blood—should be between 4.6 and 6.2 million/mm³.

reduce 1. to make smaller. 2. to lower the measured volume or weight of something. 3. restore to the original position, as in fractured bone.

referral a process by which a woman, baby or family is introduced to additional or more specialised healthcare.

referred pain pain that is felt in a different part of the body to the area of pathology.

reflex a backward or return flow of energy.

reflex action an involuntary movement which happens in response to a stimulus, e.g. light shone into the eye causes the pupil to contract.

reflexology a method of treating certain disorders in parts of the body by massaging the soles of the feet.

reflux abnormal backward flow or movement of a fluid.

regional anaesthesia an injection of drugs into a part of the body to prevent sensation being experienced in that area.

register a list on which participants or people with features in common are recorded, e.g. the *disability register*. The *birth register* is the list of names and details of all babies which is given to the registrar of births, marriages and deaths.

registrar a doctor who is undergoing advanced training in a particular field of medicine over several years.

regulation can be considered as legal restrictions promulgated by government authority.

regurgitation backward flow, maybe against gravity, of a fluid. In pregnancy regurgitation of the gastric juices through a weakened cardiac sphincter causes heartburn.

rehydration the replacement of fluids. Women in labour lose fluid due to high energy expenditure and should be offered fluids regularly in order to prevent the need to be rehydrated by intravenous means.

relapse the return of a disease after its apparent cessation.

relaxant a drug which causes relaxation of muscles; given during surgery or administered to control muscle spasm.

relaxation referring to a state of being at rest and applicable to the whole body or to individual muscles.

relaxin a hormone thought to cause general softening of tissues including cartilage. In pregnancy softening of the symphysis pubis may enable increased diameters of the pelvis.

releasing factor a trigger substance released from the hypothalamus which causes the pituitary to release hormones.

reliability the extent to which a test produces the same results with different researchers, observers and at different times.

REM (rapid eye movement) referring to a type of eye activity observed during sleep.

renal referring to the kidneys.

renal failure the kidney fails to function allowing toxins to remain in the blood where they will act like a poison. It is likely to occur following severe haemorrhage, eclampsia or infection.

renal threshold the point at which the kidney will function correctly. The threshold may be lower in pregnancy allowing substances to stay in the urine when they would normally have been reabsorbed, e.g. glucose.

renin an enzyme made, stored and secreted by the kidney. It is responsible for maintaining the blood pressure.

rennin an enzyme found in the stomach which causes milk to curdle and become insoluble.

repercussion ballottement, rebound of an object through a fluid.

reproduction the process by which two of a species create and nurture a future member of the same species.

reproductive organs the parts of the body involved in reproduction: ovaries, fallopian tubes, uterus, vagina, vulva and breasts in females; penis, testes, scrotum, prostate gland and connecting tubules in males.

research the systematic search for new knowledge.

resect removal of body tissue by surgery.

residual urine urine remaining in the bladder after micturition. More than 100 mL residual urine can indicate dysfunction.

resilience the ability of the body to return to its previous form after being stretched, as in childbirth.

resistance a force exerted against another force, usually referring to the body's ability to overcome bacterial or other infection.

resistant capacity of a microbe not to be affected by an antibiotic drug.

respectful maternity care the provision of maternity care that respects the rights of women and newborns and encompasses the right to dignity, informed consent and freedom from discrimination.

respiration breathing; the taking in of oxygen and excretion of carbon dioxide from the blood so that oxygen can be passed around the body to enable metabolism. *Artificial respiration* is a mechanical process of gaseous exchange performed when a person is unable to breathe for themselves. The lungs are inflated mechanically by a ventilator. The machine mixes gases, and monitors input and output.

respiration rate the adult average is 20 breaths per minute, while neonates vary between 40 and 60 breaths per minute.

respiratory alkalosis decreased excretion of carbon dioxide causing accumulation in the blood and altering the pH value.

respiratory arrest cessation of breathing; may be due to drugs, allergy or obstruction of the airway.

respiratory centre the area of the brain which controls the rate and depth of breathing.

respiratory distress syndrome (RDS) a condition mostly seen in preterm infants caused by lack of surfactant. Lung expansion cannot be maintained, and oxygen and CO_2 exchange is impaired. The baby becomes exhausted by the efforts of breathing and there is characteristic flaring of the nares, expiratory grunt, sternal and intercostal recession.

respiratory tract the interconnecting structures of the nose, bronchus, bronchioles, trachea, pharynx and lungs by means of which air enters the body ready for gaseous exchange.

respiratory tract infection any infection of the upper respiratory tract (e.g. sinusitis, laryngitis, tonsillitis) or the lower respiratory tract (e.g. bronchitis, pneumonia).

restitution returning to the correct place. The fetal head immediately after delivery rotates to restore alignment with the shoulders.

resuscitation restoration from a state of collapse. *Neonatal resuscitation* is necessary for infants who fail to breathe spontaneously at birth.

retained placenta describes the situation where the placenta has not been delivered within what is deemed a locally appropriate time after the delivery of the baby. It may need to be removed manually.

retching attempting to be sick.

retention holding on to, holding back. In *urinary retention* the bladder fails to evacuate urine.

reticular resembling a net in form.

reticuloendothelial system a network of cells found in the connective tissue, lungs, liver, spleen and bone marrow. They are concerned with the formation and destruction of red blood cells (erythrocytes), storage of fats, storage of iron, inflammation and immunity. Some cells move in the blood and can ingest foreign materials.

retina the inner lining of the eye which receives light images and sends them to the brain for interpretation.

retinal detachment the retina comes away from the choroids. Further detachment may occur if women with this condition push vigorously during the second stage of labour. They may choose assisted delivery or prefer to adopt upright positions which enable the baby to be born without vigorous pushing.

retinopathy refers to damage to the retina.

retinopathy of prematurity iatrogenic retinal opacity and occlusion occurring secondary to oxygen therapy which has been given to the premature newborn.

retracted nipple a nipple which is drawn inwards by fibrotic bands of tissue beneath the skin and does not protrude easily even when stimulated.

retraction pulling back. A state of permanent shortening of uterine muscle fibres

occurring during contraction.
Following relaxation some of
the shortening is retained.
The next contraction requires
less effort to achieve the same
traction achieving a state of
progressive dilation.

retractor a surgical instrument
used to pull back another
organ from the field of
operation.

retro- combining form
meaning behind or at
the back.

retroflexion the bending of an
organ or part so that its top is
turned posteriorly. A
retroflexion of the uterus is
where the body of the uterus
is turned towards the cervix,
resulting in a sharp angle at
the point of bending.

retrograde moving backwards.

retrograde menstruation the
backflow of the menstrual
discharge through the uterus,
fallopian tubes and into the
abdominal cavity.

retroplacental behind the
placenta.

retroplacental clot a collection
of blood behind the placenta.

retroversion bending
backwards.

retroversion of the uterus
refers to the whole uterus
being bent or tilted
backwards instead of
forwards (*see* Fig. 84).

retroverted gravid uterus
when a retroverted uterus
containing a pregnancy
becomes trapped in the
pelvis, its passage being
obstructed by the sacral
promontory.

retrovirus a group of RNA
viruses including the ones
causing HIV. These viruses
replicate by inserting a DNA
copy of their genome into a
healthy host cell.

Rh factor an antigen which
may be present or absent on
the red cells causing the
blood group to be termed
Rh-negative or Rh-positive;
previously called rhesus
factor.

**Rh immune globulin (Rh(D)
immunoglobulin)** the
immune globulin which is
offered to Rh-negative
mothers during pregnancy,
after miscarriage, termination
of pregnancy or birth unless
the infant is also Rh-negative.
It can prevent the mother
developing antibodies to the
Rh positive factor which may
pass into her circulation
during placental separation.
The immunoglobulin coats
the fetal blood cells so
that the mother's body does
not recognise them as foreign
proteins.

Rh incompatibility the
mismatch between two
groups of blood cells—
mother and fetus or donor
to recipient's blood. The
Rh factor is present in the
blood of one but not
the other so agglutination
(sticking together of the
cells) can occur if fetal blood
escapes into the maternal
circulation.

rheumatism a common term
for a number of inflammatory
or connective tissue disorders

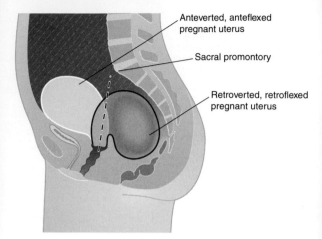

Anteverted, anteflexed pregnant uterus

Sacral promontory

Retroverted, retroflexed pregnant uterus

Figure 84
Retroversion of the uterus

especially those that affect the joints.

rhinitis inflammation of the mucous membrane of the nose.

rhomboid of Michaelis a diamond-shaped area that can be seen on the buttocks (*see* Fig. 85).

rhythm a constantly repeating sequence of events.

rhythm method of family planning a method of avoiding pregnancy based on avoiding intercourse during the ovulatory phase of the menstrual cycle. It is dependent on a predictable cycle, and a record of past cycles. This method may also be combined with observation of the basal body temperature and the texture of the vaginal secretions in order to establish the 'safe' period for sexual intercourse.

ribonucleic acid (RNA) the cytoplasmic acid found in cells which translate the DNA information into action.

rickets deformity of the bones caused by dietary lack of vitamin D in the formative years.

right occipitoanterior (ROA) refers to the position of the

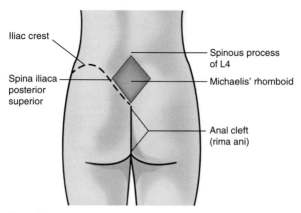

Figure 85
Rhomboid of Michaelis
Illustration by Alan Laver

fetal skull in relation to the maternal pelvis. The back of the head, the occiput, is positioned to the front and right side of the maternal pelvis.

right occipitolateral (ROL) the fetal occiput in utero is to the right side of the maternal pelvis.

right occipitoposterior (ROP) the occiput is on the right side and to the back of the maternal pelvis.

right sacroanterior (RSA) refers to the position of the fetus when the breech is presenting. The sacrum (the bony eminence above the buttocks) is to the front right side of the mother's pelvis.

right sacrolateral (RSL) when the breech is presenting and the sacrum is on the right and to the side of the mother's pelvis.

right sacroposterior (RSP) when the breech is presenting and the sacrum is on the right side and the back of the mother's pelvis.

right-to-left shunt an abnormal communication/hole between the atria which enables passage of blood from one side to the other.

rigor an attack of shivering and shaking seen in response to a rise in the body temperature.

risk factor a factor in the health or history of an individual which may make them more susceptible to a specific complication occurring. Risk factors in pregnancy include certain medical and previous obstetric conditions.

risk management a structure designed to identify and eliminate risks ensuring optimal care and preventing medical and legal problems. A process of assessing risks and developing strategies to coordinate the prevention and management of those risks.

Ritter's disease a severe form of pemphigus neonatorum. A staphylococcal skin infection.

rockerbottom feet (congenital vertical talus) a rare rigid deformity of the feet. Such an anomaly may suggest a chromosomal abnormality such as trisomy 18.

role an exhibited pattern of behaviour enacted to fulfil a given expectation.

role conflict the presence of contradictory elements within one's expected behaviour.

role model a person whose action inspires another to similar behaviour.

rooming-in a system in which the baby remains at the mother's bedside throughout its stay in hospital.

rooting reflex the innate ability of the neonate to search for and find the nipple.

roseola a pink/rose-coloured rash.

rotation turning round. Refers to the ability of the fetal head

when deep in the pelvis to be deflected by the pelvic floor muscles so that it turns round to accommodate itself to the shape of the outlet.

rotavirus a wheel-shaped virus that causes diarrhoea in infants.

roughage the indigestible parts of the diet which pass through the intestines encouraging peristalsis.

round ligament a sheet of tissue extending from the cornua of the uterus to the vulva (*see* Fig. 86).

RU 486 (mifepristone) progesterone receptor antagonist that dilates the cervix and sensitises the myometrium to the effects of prostaglandins. It is given orally and used for the medical termination of first or second trimester pregnancy.

rubella (SYNONYM German measles) a viral infection with symptoms of the common cold and macular rash. If it occurs in the first trimester of pregnancy it can cause congenital anomaly of the heart, eye or ear or even stillbirth. Vaccination against rubella is offered at 12 months with the MMR vaccine (measles, mumps, rubella) and again at 18 months with the MMRV vaccine (measles, mumps, rubella, varicella). Vaccination schedules may differ between countries.

Rubins 1 an external manoeuvre used to manage

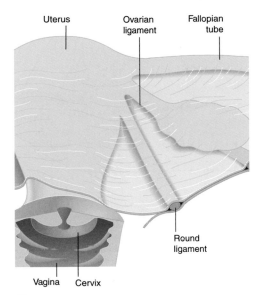

Uterus · Ovarian ligament · Fallopian tube

Round ligament

Vagina · Cervix

Figure 86
Round ligament

shoulder dystocia. Suprapubic pressure is applied to the woman's abdomen over where the baby's anterior shoulder would be to make the shoulder fold forwards, reducing the bisacromial diameter and allowing the baby to be born (*see* Fig. 87).

Rubins 2 an internal manoeuvre used to manage shoulder dystocia usually undertaken when Rubins 1 is unsuccessful. The fingers of the accoucheur are inserted into the woman's vagina and the baby's anterior shoulder is rotated forwards, reducing the bisacromial diameter and allowing the baby to be born.

rugae (SINGULAR ruga) the folds or creases found in the stomach and in the vaginal wall which allow it to stretch.

rupture tearing or bursting of a tube, membrane or organ

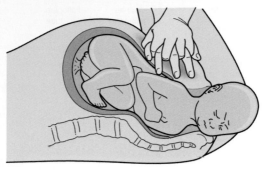

Figure 87
Rubins 1
Illustration by Alan Laver

such that the contents escape. For example, *rupture of membranes* in labour or *rupture of the uterus* in obstructed labour.

rupture of the uterus the muscle fibres of the uterus divide with loss of integrity of the cavity, displacement and likely death of the fetus, and excessive bleeding and shock in the mother.

ruptured hymen the fragmented membranous tags found in the vagina indicative of penetrative intercourse.

Ss

Sabin vaccine three live but weakened polio viruses which are given orally in an attempt to enable the body to develop its own immunity to polio.

sac pouch or pocket-like cavity.

sacculation of the uterus a term applied to the incarcerated gravid uterus. The rise of the uterus into the abdominal cavity is obstructed by the sacral promontory. Only the anterior aspect of the uterus will grow with stretching of the urethra and causing retention of urine.

sacral, sacro- referring to the sacrum.

sacral promontory the anterior aspect of the first sacral vertebra which protrudes into the pelvic inlet and is a featured landmark.

sacral vertebrae the five bones of the spinal column which fuse together to form the sacrum and posterior aspect of the pelvis. They have a convex anterior surface.

sacrococcygeal refers to the sacrum and the coccyx.

sacrocotyloid referring to the sacrum and the acetabulum. The distance is occasionally measured and should be 9.5 cm otherwise a contracted pelvis may be suspected.

sacroiliac refers to the sacrum and the ilium.

sacroiliac joint the fixed joint between the ilium and the sacrum which might be slightly movable in pregnancy.

sacrum large wedge-shaped bone composed of five fused vertebrae situated at the lower end of the spinal column and forming the back wall of the pelvic girdle.

safe sex the practice of using condoms during sexual intercourse to prevent the exchange of bodily fluids thereby preventing the possible transmission of diseases including the HIV virus.

Safer Baby Bundle a collection of interventions being implemented in Australia to reduce late pregnancy stillbirth.

sagittal an imaginary line extending from the front to the back of the body and bisecting a region, referred to as a sagittal section. The *sagittal suture* is a suture separating the parietal bones.

sagittal fontanelle a soft area on the sagittal suture posterior to the bregma. It may be found in some neonates and babies with Down syndrome.

salicylate a salt found in preparations such as aspirin used as an antipyretic, anti-inflammatory and analgesic. It works by inhibiting prostaglandin manufacture which is responsible for inflammation.

saline a solution containing water and 0.9% salt.

saliva the secretions of the mouth which moisten food and start the process of carbohydrate digestion.

Salmonella bacteria responsible for causing gastroenteritis. The causative organism in several outbreaks of food poisoning with associated fatalities.

salpingectomy removal of the fallopian tube.

salpingitis inflammation of the fallopian tube.

salpingogram procedure whereby a radio contrast medium is introduced via the cervix, pumped into the uterus and X-rays are taken as it passes through the fallopian tubes into the abdomen. It is done to establish patency of the tube.

salpingography X-ray images of the fallopian tubes produced after injection of radio-opaque contrast medium.

salpingo-oophorectomy removal of the fallopian tube and ovary.

salpingotomy cutting into or opening up of the fallopian tube.

salpinx a tube, usually the fallopian tube.

salutogenesis a concept which focuses on maintaining and supporting optimal health.

sample a group in the population selected as representative of the entire population. Research will be conducted with the cooperation of the group and results will be generalised to the population.

sanguine abundant blood in the circulation giving a ruddy complexion and an attitude of vitality and confidence.

sanitary napkin (SYNONYM sanitary towel) a pad used to absorb menstrual flow. May be disposable or washable/ recyclable.

sanitation the maintenance of a healthy, disease-free environment.

SARS (severe acute respiratory syndrome) a severe respiratory illness that is caused by a coronavirus.

SARS-CoV-2 (severe acute respiratory syndrome coronavirus 2) the strain of coronavirus that causes coronavirus disease 2019 (COVID-19), the respiratory illness responsible for the COVID-19 pandemic.

scabies skin infestation with the human itch mite. It is highly contagious. The itch mite burrows just below the skin and can cause a reaction.

scalp the skin over the top of the head out of which the hair grows.

scalpel a very fine, sharp knife used for making surgical incisions (cutting).

scan an examination of a part of the body using computer-generated images to determine abnormal conditions. In *ultrasound scanning* (USS) sound waves are used to generate images of structures within the body.

scapula the flat triangular bone found behind the shoulder.

scarlet fever contagious disease of childhood caused by *haemolytic Streptococcus A*. Typical presentation is a red rash, fever, sore throat, headache and vomiting.

scavenger system a system designed to remove anaesthetic gases from the air.

schedule of drugs a means of categorising drugs according to their potential for abuse.

schizophrenia mental health disorder that affects a person's ability to think, feel and act.

Schultze expulsion of the placenta the fetal surface of the placenta appears first at the vulva during the third stage of labour, as opposed to the maternal surface (*see* Matthew Duncan expulsion and Fig. 88).

sciatic nerve a nerve which runs down the back of the leg from the spine.

sciatica severe pain which results from compression of the sciatic nerve. It follows the pathway of a nerve.

scientific method a systematic, ordered way of collecting information in order to formulate theory and predict relationships.

sclerema hardening of the skin and subcutaneous tissue.

sclerema neonatorum subcutaneous hardening of the tissues of the extremities, often due to hypothermia in newborn infants.

scoliosis curving of the spine, also known as lordosis or kyphosis.

screening a test which can be carried out on a large

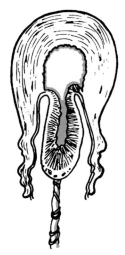

Figure 88
Schultze expulsion of the placenta

population of apparently healthy people in order to attempt to detect and thus treat diseases early. The test has to be acceptable, reliable (not too many false-positives or false-negatives) and cost-effective. There is a clear distinction between a screening test, which can give an indication of the likelihood of existence of disease, and a diagnostic test, which can positively detect a disease.

scrotum the sac behind the penis in which the testes are located.

scurvy a disease caused by lack of vitamin C in the diet. The person becomes anaemic, develops mouth ulcers, haemorrhages into the mucous membranes and the skin, and has swollen, painful joints.

sebaceous oily.

sebaceous glands small, oil-producing glands near the surface of the skin.

sebum the oily substance produced by the sebaceous glands.

second degree perineal laceration damage to the pelvic floor, including the perineal skin and muscle layers, sustained during the birth of a baby.

second stage of labour the period of labour from the complete dilation of the cervix until the complete birth of the infant. It lasts from several minutes up to 3 or more hours.

secondary an event which occurs after the main event; not the primary event.

secondary areola development of an extended pigmented area around the areola occurring in pregnancy.

secondary postpartum haemorrhage excessive bleeding from the genital tract commencing 24 hours and up to 6 weeks after birth of the baby, usually due to infection or retained products of conception.

secretion a substance produced by a gland.

secretory phase the second half of the menstrual cycle, after the ovum has been released approximately 14 days before the menses.

The corpus luteum increases production of progesterone bringing about glandular activity in the endometrium and a receptive state for the fertilised ovum (*see* Fig. 89).

sedative a drug given to induce deep relaxation and reduce anxiety.

segment a part of the whole. *Upper segment of the uterus*—the body of the uterus responsible for contracting and thickening in labour. *Lower segment of the uterus*—the lower third of the uterus and the cervix, which relaxes and dilates in labour.

segmentation the process of dividing the whole into parts similar to the whole.

seizure a convulsion or epileptic fit.

self-awareness the development of understanding of one's own beliefs, biases, previous experiences and attitudes and conscious insight into how these can affect one's philosophy and approach to people and practice.

self-concept the image of self, including attitudes that a person holds in their mind.

self-conscious being aware of oneself and one's likely reactions, feelings and desires.

self-esteem the degree of worth one attributes to oneself.

self-help group a collection of people with similar interests who meet together to discuss and support one another.

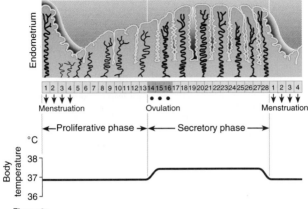

Figure 89
Secretory phase

Sellick's manoeuvre the procedure of applying pressure on the cricoid cartilage of the larynx to occlude the oesophagus in order to prevent regurgitation of stomach contents during intubation.

semen the fluid from the prostate gland containing sperm which is ejaculated from the penis during intercourse.

semi- prefix meaning half or partial.

semiconscious a state in which the person is not fully alert or aware of their surroundings.

semipermeable allowing some substances through but not all. The placenta and membranes are semipermeable, allowing some viruses, drugs and alcohol to pass through to the fetus.

semiprone lying on one side with the topmost thigh and arm flexed and forward.

semirecumbent reclining position, half sitting up.

senile vaginitis age-related degeneration of the vagina in which the tissues become less vascular, less elastic and dryer; may occur postmenopausally as the levels of oestrogen secretion fall.

sensation a feeling, impression or awareness of one's physical and emotional state.

sensitisation an immunological response occurring after initial exposure of a person to an antigen. The preparation of an organ (e.g. the uterus) by bathing it in a hormone such as prostaglandin so that it will respond to another hormone such as oxytocin, triggering contraction and the start of labour.

sensitive reacting to a stimulus.

sensory referring to the senses or sensation.

sensory nerves nerves that detect pressure, pain and temperature and relay this stimulus to the brain for interpretation.

sentinel event a serious unanticipated event in a healthcare setting that is not related to the natural course of the patient's illness resulting in death or serious physical or psychological injury.

separation anxiety the stress symptoms exhibited by an infant when removed from her or his mother or main carer or when approached by a stranger.

sepsis infection; the presence of harmful organisms where they can cause tissue damage. *Puerperal sepsis* is infection of the genital tract after delivery.

sepsis 6 refers to six steps to be delivered in 1 hour to reduce mortality in patients with sepsis: blood cultures, check full blood count and lactate, IV fluid, IV antibiotics, monitor urine output and give oxygen. Also known as sepsis bundle or sepsis pathway.

septal defect a congenital abnormality in the wall which divides the left and right sides of the heart, frequently a fistula.

septic the presence of infection.

septic abortion an abortion following which an infection occurs in the uterus, sometimes due to the use of unclean instruments. It can be life-threatening.

septicaemia bacteria in the blood. The person will be very ill, with pyrexia, nausea, vomiting, rigors, headache, joint pains and general malaise.

septum an anatomical structure which divides an organ or tube in half. The left and right side of the heart are divided by a septum. An unusual uterine anomaly is a septum descending from the fundus which may go through to the vagina or terminate just below the fundus forming a bicornuate uterus.

septuplets seven babies in the uterus or being born at the same time.

sequela (PLURAL sequelae) that which follows or results from something. Referring to a lifelong condition which may follow and be caused by childbirth.

seroconversion the change seen in a series of blood/serology tests, such as antibodies developing in response to a vaccine or infection.

serology the use of antigen/antibody reactions in the laboratory to diagnose infection in blood taken from clients.

serous fluid any fluid resembling serum.

serous membrane a thin but strong sheet of cells which lines cavities. The thoracic and abdominal cavities are lined by two such membranes between which serous fluid is produced, enabling the membranes to move against each other without friction.

serum the yellow sticky fluid left when the cells have been removed from blood.

serum albumin one of the main proteins in the blood which is responsible for its viscosity and maintenance of blood pressure.

serum bilirubin (SBR) the presence in the blood of bilirubin, the product of red cell (erythrocyte) breakdown. Found in the blood of neonates with physiological jaundice. The level is monitored by taking blood from a heel prick and phototherapy is offered if levels are high. High levels can cause staining of the medulla of the brain—kernicterus—and irreversible damage.

sex (gender) species are divided into male and female depending on which gametes they have.

sex chromosome termed the X and Y chromosomes; the genetic component in determining gender.

sex hormones endocrine hormones such as androgens and oestrogens produced by the testes or ovaries that are responsible for influencing development of sexual characteristics.

sexism behavioural characteristics of prejudice or discriminatory belief that one gender is superior to another.

sex-linked genes refers to the genes which are found only on the sex chromosomes. Some diseases are sex-linked (e.g. haemophilia).

sextuplets six babies in the uterus or being born at the same time.

sexual abuse the forcing upon a person of sexual acts or practices against their will and without their consensual participation.

sexual health freedom from sexually transmitted infection and ability to enjoy sexual expression.

sexual intercourse the physical process during which the erect penis is introduced into the vagina and semen is ejaculated. Sperm in the semen are able to pass through the cervix and swim towards the fallopian tubes in search of an ovum with which to unite.

sexually transmitted infection (STI) diseases such as infection with *Chlamydia trachomatis*, HIV, syphilis and gonorrhoea, which can be passed on during sexual intercourse.

shaken baby syndrome a severe form of head injury caused by violently shaking an infant or child.

shared care a system whereby the woman receives antenatal care in a collaborative format both from the midwife and from a doctor in a hospital or other clinical setting.

shared decision-making involves the integration of a woman's values, goals and concerns with the best available evidence about benefits, risks and uncertainties of treatment, in order to achieve appropriate healthcare decisions. It involves clinicians and the woman making decisions together about the woman's management.

sharps used scalpels and needles which are able to cause a laceration or puncture wound and possibly transmit disease to the injured person.

sheath (SYNONYM condom) the rubber tube which is put over the erect penis before penetration during sexual intercourse. It prevents the sperm entering the female body and so avoids conception.

Sheehan's syndrome hypoxia and pituitary necrosis following severe intrapartum conditions such as abruptio placentae or postpartum haemorrhage which can cause shock. Pituitary function is impaired and secondary infertility may ensue.

Shirodkar operation surgical procedure performed at around 16 weeks' gestation where the cervix is deemed 'incompetent'. A purse-string suture is put around the neck of the cervix to keep it closed and in an attempt to prevent abortion.

Shirodkar suture the purse-string suture which is inserted into the cervix during a Shirodkar operation.

shivering involuntary contraction of the tiny muscles under the skin in order to generate heat when cold or in response to fear.

shock a physical state characterised by sudden fall in blood pressure, rapid pulse, abnormal breathing patterns, pallor and loss of full consciousness. Severe shock can be potentially life-threatening.

shoulder dystocia an emergency situation occasionally occurring in the second stage of labour. The head of the baby is born and no further advance takes place as the shoulders fail to rotate, descend and deliver; the anterior shoulder is impacted behind the symphysis pubis.

shoulder presentation the shoulder is presenting over the cervix (see Fig. 90). This is incompatible with vaginal

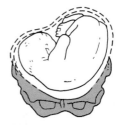

Figure 90
Shoulder presentation

birth and labour is obstructed. A caesarean section is usually offered on diagnosis.

show (SYNONYM operculum) the mucus plug expelled from the cervical canal as the cervix starts to efface and dilate.

shunt the rerouting or bypassing of an organ by an abnormal anatomical opening, e.g. the ductus arteriosus causes blood to bypass the lungs.

SI units (Système International d'Unités; International System of Units) an internationally agreed scale of measurement used in science, industry and pharmaceuticals. It uses metres, kilograms and seconds. (*See* Appendix 2.)

Siamese twins (SYNONYM conjoined twins) incomplete cleavage of a single fertilised ovum; two babies develop but are anatomically joined at some point.

siblings one, two or more children having the same parents; blood relatives.

sickle cell anaemia a chronic incurable anaemia caused by homozygosity to haemoglobin S. The abnormal haemoglobin makes the erythrocytes very fragile and susceptible to alteration in shape, sometimes triggering a sickle cell crisis.

sickle cell crisis alteration in the shape of erythrocytes when the tension (concentration) of oxygen in the cells falls. They are unable to absorb as much oxygen. The loss of discoid shape causes the cells to clump or stick together and so obstruct blood vessels resulting

in ischaemia. Severe joint pain, headaches, dizziness, convulsions, visual disturbances, facial nerve paralysis, breathlessness, cyanosis and shock may result.

sickle cell disease a disease caused by abnormally shaped erythrocytes. Sickle cell crises will occur when the person is stressed. Anaemia is common.

sickle cell trait the haemoglobin S gene has been inherited from one parent. The carrier may have some haemoglobin S but no signs or symptoms of the disease.

side effect a secondary and undesirable reaction accompanying the desired effect of a drug given with therapeutic intent.

SIDS *see* sudden infant death syndrome.

sigmoid S-shaped region of the large intestine/colon.

sign an indication; something visible, objective.

significance having an uncertainty of meaning; statistical probability that a given finding may have occurred by chance alone.

silver nitrate an anti-infective agent historically used in eye drops to prevent gonococcal ophthalmia neonatorum.

Simmonds' disease hypoactivity of the pituitary gland causing all other endocrine glands to be underactive.

sinciput the brow or the forehead of the fetus; the region found between the coronal suture and orbital ridges.

singleton denotes the presence of a single fetus in the uterus throughout pregnancy.

skeletal system the combined structure of bones and cartilage providing the protective frame and structure for the body and enabling movement.

Skene's ducts the largest of the urethral glands in the female. They provide lubrication and are equated to the prostate gland in the male.

skull the bony cap over the top of the brain. It comprises three regions: the vault, the face and the base.

small for gestational age (SGA) a baby that is smaller than expected for its gestation. Detection (by palpation and ultrasound) is important because the fetus is at risk of hypoxia in labour and postnatal problems.

smear a small sample of superficial cells which are removed from the cervix to detect hormonal levels and early malignant changes.

smegma the sebaceous secretion that accumulates around the glans penis and the clitoris.

social network a grouping of people with common interests who willingly interact together with mutual benefits.

social services department the government department which is concerned with the welfare of low-income families and those with special needs, disabilities and long-term diseases. Also known as department of community services in some countries.

social worker a person trained to assess social need and direct people to appropriate resources. There is a responsibility towards vulnerable members of society, children, the elderly and the homeless.

socioeconomic status the position of an individual on a scale determined by wealth, health and education.

sociology the study of society and how it functions.

soft chancre (SYNONYM chancroid) a lesion of the genitalia, usually of venereal origin, caused by *Haemophilus ducreyi*.

soft palate (SYNONYM velum, muscular palate) the soft tissue constituting the back of the roof of the mouth and not containing bone.

solar plexus network of nerves and ganglia in the peritoneal cavity behind the stomach that supplies nerves to the abdominal viscera.

somersault maneuver a technique used to manage a nuchal cord during birth.

sonogram the image obtained by ultrasound scan.

sonography ultrasonography.

souffle a soft blowing sound heard over the abdomen in pregnancy. A *uterine souffle* is the pulsating sound of the uterine arteries.

Spalding's sign the overlapping of the bones of the cranium seen on X-ray examination after fetal death.

spasm an involuntary and uncontrollable movement in a muscle. It is not under the control of the brain.

spastic refers to limb movements which are not under the control of the will/brain. Usually due to cerebral palsy.

special care baby unit (SCBU), special care nursery (SCN) a department set up with equipment and staff to care for the particular needs of babies born preterm or otherwise in poor health. They can sometimes have an intensive care unit attached which specialises in babies needing ventilation.

specific gravity refers to the weight of a fluid compared to water using the same volume. The specific gravity of water is 1.00 while urine may be 1.010 or more depending on its concentration.

specimen a small sample of the whole; tests can be performed on samples to diagnose the wellbeing of the whole.

speculum an instrument used to inspect a cavity not usually visible, e.g. the cervix can be seen by inserting a speculum in the vagina.

Spencer Wells artery forceps a type of artery forceps used in surgical procedures.

spermatic referring to sperm.

spermatic cord comprises arteries, nerves and the tube along which sperm pass from the testes to reach the penis.

spermatogenesis the differentiation of spermatogonial cells (primordial germ cells in the testes) into spermatozoa.

spermatozoa mature reproductive cells. They are 50 μm (micrometres) long, have a head with a nucleus, a neck and a tail for propulsion (*see* Fig. 91).

spermicide a cream or gel which is destructive to sperm.

sphincter a strong, round band of muscle fibres which closes or opens a tube or cavity, e.g. the *pyloric sphincter*, the *cardiac sphincter* in the stomach, or the *anal sphincter* which closes the rectum.

sphingomyelin a complex molecule of fat and protein found in the amniotic fluid and measured as a comparative ratio to lecithin to assess fetal lung maturity.

sphygmomanometer an instrument used to measure blood pressure.

spina bifida congenital abnormality of the central nervous system. The bony cavity around the spinal cord is not completely closed and so the meninges herniate through. In severe cases the spinal cord is partially exposed (*see* Fig. 92).

spinal refers to the spine.

spinal anaesthetic (SYNONYM spinal block) the dura around the spinal cord is pierced and local anaesthetic is introduced into the cerebrospinal fluid. The sensory nerves are

From above

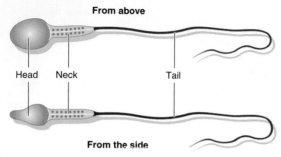

Head   Neck   Tail

From the side

Figure 91
Spermatozoa

blocked for a short period of time.

spinal headache a severe headache following an epidural anaesthetic, lumbar puncture or spinal block caused by the escape of cerebrospinal fluid during the procedure. The headache and accompanying visual disturbances may last several days.

spine the bones of the back that make up the vertebrae and enclose the spinal cord.

spinous process small projections of bony tissue found mainly on the spinal column.

spirochaete a group of microorganisms which appear spiral under a microscope; they cause syphilis.

spirometer an instrument for measuring the air inhaled into and exhaled out of the lungs, such as in pulmonary function tests.

splanchnic pertaining to the viscera.

spleen a large, lymphatic organ that is left of the stomach below the diaphragm. It is important for the storage of blood, disintegration of old blood cells, filtering of foreign substances from the blood, and producing lymphocytes.

splint a solid board used to hold the joints either side of a fracture in place or to immobilise an arm if there is an intravenous infusion in place.

spondylosis degeneration of the spinal column, especially a fusion and immobilisation of the vertebral bones.

spontaneous resulting from natural impulses; happening without intervention.

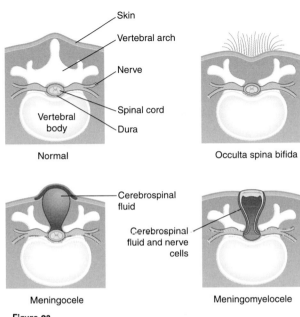

Figure 92
Spina bifida

spontaneous labour the birthing process from the beginning to the end without recourse to mechanical or pharmacological help.

spontaneous miscarriage the natural loss of a pregnancy before it is viable.

spontaneous vaginal birth (SVB) normal birth of a baby through the vagina.

spurious labour a false labour.

squamous epithelium the thin fish-like scaly appearance of the cells lining the mouth and vagina.

squatting a position adopted for birth in which the woman crouches close to the ground. A variation of this is the supported squat in which the woman stands with her hips and knees completely flexed supporting herself on her arms or being supported by another. The dimensions of the pelvic outlet are enlarged.

standard a measure which forms the basis of other similar phenomena, values, substances or against which they can be compared or judged. A standard is a predetermined criterion or description of care, used to provide guidance, and can be a measure by which high-quality care and professional performance are assessed.

standard deviation a mathematical statement used to describe the dispersion of a set of values or scores from the mean value or score. Each value is subtracted from the mean, squared and the squares are summed. The square root of the summed squares gives a mathematically standardised value so that deviations in the sample can be compared.

standard of care written statement explaining what a person can expect from the professionals around them and by which the professional's performance can be measured.

staphylococci (SINGULAR staphylococcus) a group of pus-forming bacteria which look like a bunch of grapes under a microscope; they can cause puerperal sepsis,

urinary tract infections, skin infections and sore throats.

staples small U-shaped pieces of wire used to hold the edges of a skin wound together after surgery and until healing has occurred.

startle reflex (SYNONYM Moro reflex) an involuntary spasmodic movement of the limbs of the infant in response to a sudden stimulus. Used to assess neonates. The head is allowed to drop back; the arms will swing out and return to their midline flexed position in a series of jerks. Disturbance in the pattern may indicate neurological damage.

stasis loss of peristaltic movement. *Intestinal stasis* causes constipation and after surgery paralytic ileus (in which the gut is temporarily paralysed).

stat. (LATIN *statim*) abbreviation used in prescribing medicines meaning given at once, immediately.

station refers to the position of the fetal head in relation to the ischial spine (*see* Fig. 93). It can be assessed on vaginal examination.

statistical significance the interpretation of data suggesting that results arose from a known factor and not simply by chance.

statistics figures and numbers which lead to the postulation of facts and theories.

status epilepticus a rapid succession of epileptic fits

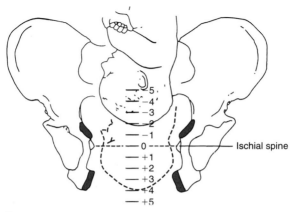

Figure 93
Stations of the fetal head

with no time for recovery between.

statutory referring to legislation by parliament.

Stein-Leventhal syndrome a group of symptoms including amenorrhoea, oligomenorrhoea, hirsutism, infertility, polycystic ovaries and high levels of testosterone.

stem cells master cells which develop a few days after fertilisation of the ovum. They contain enzymes which enable rapid cell replication and have the capacity to develop into many different specialised tissue cells, e.g. blood, skin, muscle, nerves, etc.

stenosis narrowing, contraction, usually of a muscle. *Pyloric stenosis* is when the sphincter muscle which closes the lower part of the stomach hardens and food cannot pass through. This may be congenital. Surgical correction will be offered.

stereotype a particular view, belief or assumption attributed to a person or group of people based on external characteristics.

sterile 1. unable to conceive children. 2. without the presence of microorganisms or spores.

sterile water injections (SWI) are an effective method for the relief of back pain in labour. The procedure involves a small amount of sterile water injected under the skin at four locations on the lower back (sacrum).

sterilisation 1. the process by which an object becomes totally free from microbes. 2. surgical procedure to ligate the fallopian tubes or the vas deferens (vasectomy) so that fertilisation cannot occur.

sternum bone at the centre front of the ribs, the breast bone.

steroids a group of different hormones with the same basic chemical structure produced mainly by the adrenal cortex and the gonads. Artificially administered, they are used to reduce inflammation not caused by infection.

stethoscope an instrument with earpieces and tubule for amplification used to auscultate the heart and other sounds within the body. A fetal stethoscope is a trumpet-shaped instrument which when placed over the maternal abdomen will detect the sound of the fetal heart.

stillbirth baby who is born without any signs of life at or after 20 weeks of pregnancy (in some countries, 24 weeks is used as the cut-off).

stimulate to bring about action. The healthcare professional may stimulate a newborn infant to breathe for the first time.

stimulus anything which causes a person or an organ to respond or become more active than previously; may refer to some drugs.

stomach the sac-like structure at the end of the oesophagus just below the diaphragm into which food passes after being swallowed and in which further digestion occurs.

stool discharge from the rectum.

strabismus a squint, a congenital abnormality of the eyes. One eye appears to look one way while the other eye looks elsewhere.

straight sinus a blood vessel found at the junction of the falx cerebri and the tentorium cerebelli within the skull (*see* Fig. 94). In conditions associated with abnormal moulding of the fetal skull it may rupture causing internal haemorrhage and resultant morbidity or mortality.

strawberry mark a congenital mark that is generally red and caused by a cluster of capillaries near the surface of the skin. It usually fades.

streptococcus (PLURAL streptococci) small, round-shaped bacteria common in the environment and harboured in the throat and nose. Some strains like beta-haemolytic streptococci can cause scarlet fever, tonsillitis and severe puerperal sepsis.

stress tension of the body or mind. If the tension is

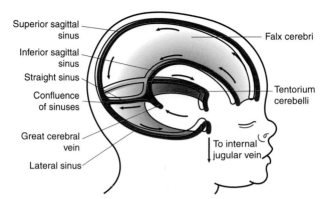

Figure 94
Straight sinus

---

excessive or prolonged,
physical or mental
dysfunction will occur.
striae gravidarum ('stretch
marks') marks over the
abdomen, breasts and thighs
which can develop during
pregnancy as the collagen
fibres in the skin tear. They
are red at first and fade to
silver.
strip membranes vaginal
examination whereby a finger
is inserted through the
cervical os and the amnion
and chorion are separated
from the lower segment of the
uterus. This may stimulate the
release of oxytocin and
prostaglandins and initiate the
start of labour.
sub- prefix meaning beneath,
under or below.

subarachnoid below the
arachnoid mater (membrane),
one of the meninges lining
the brain and spinal cord.
subarachnoid haemorrhage
bleeding into the
subarachnoid space.
subarachnoid space not a real
space but the area between
the arachnoid and the pia
mater in which the
cerebrospinal fluid circulates.
subclavian beneath the clavicle.
subclavian artery main artery
which supplies blood to the
arm.
subcutaneous under the skin,
into the tissue below the skin.
subcutaneous adipose tissue
the fat deposits under the
skin.
subcuticular suture a method
of bringing together two

surfaces by placing a continuous suture beneath the skin along the whole length of the wound. It cannot be seen on the surface and may be more comfortable for the woman than intermittent sutures.

subdural under the dura mater (the membrane surrounding the brain and spinal cord).

subdural haemorrhage bleeding under the dura mater; also called intracranial haemorrhage. Usually results from a traumatic instrumental delivery.

subfertility failure to conceive after unprotected sexual intercourse for more than 1 year (some jurisdictions 6 months).

subinvolution delay in return of the uterus to its non-pregnant size. This may be due to retained products, infection or caesarean section.

subjective information or experiences as perceived by one person.

sublingual refers to the area under the tongue. A drug can be placed under the tongue where it dissolves and is absorbed by the mucous membranes.

subluxation partial dislocation of a joint or occasionally a ligament.

submucous under the mucous membrane.

subnormal less than that expected of the majority of the population.

submentobregmatic presenting diameter of the fetal skull in a fully extended face presentation. Measured from the junction of chin and neck to the middle point of the anterior fontanelle and measures 9.5 cm (*see* Fig. 95).

suboccipitobregmatic a measurement of the fetal head taken from just above the neck posteriorly to the bregma or anterior fontanelle. It is the smallest diameter and presents when the head is well flexed (*see* Fig. 95).

subtotal hysterectomy removal of the body of the uterus, but the cervix and ovaries remain.

succenturiate additional, accessory.

succenturiate placenta (SYNONYM accessory lobe) placenta containing an extra lobe which is not part of the main organ but is supplied with blood from vessels running through the membranes. The lobe can become detached from the main placenta during the third stage of labour and may possibly remain in the uterus contributing to infection or potentially causing haemorrhage (*see* Fig. 76).

suck to draw into the mouth by creating a vacuum and negative pressure with the lips and tongue.

sucking blister formation of a small callous pad on the upper or lower lip of a baby which develops after sucking. It may resemble a blister.

sucking reflex the inborn ability of the newborn to suck in response to stimulation.

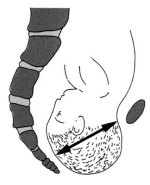 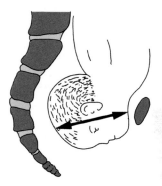

Suboccipitobregmatic 9.5 cm
vertex presentation

Submentobregmatic 9.5 cm
face presentation

Figure 95
Suboccipitobregmatic presentations

sudden infant death syndrome (SIDS) death of a healthy infant for no apparent cause. Most common between the age of 3 weeks and 6 months and occurring mainly at night; so-called 'cot death'. *See also* sudden unexpected death in infancy (SUDI).

sudden unexpected death in infancy (SUDI) a term used when a sudden and unexpected death of a baby occurs and the cause of the death is not immediately apparent. Sudden infant death syndrome (SIDS) is a subset of SUDI and the term is only used when no cause of death is found.

sulcus a groove, fold or furrow as between cotyledons of the placenta.

sulfonamides a group of chemicals with a sulfur base used to treat infections especially streptococci, gonococci and *E. coli*.

super-, supra- prefixes meaning over, above or on top of.

superfecundation extra abundant fertility; the fertilisation of two ova within the same ovulatory cycle by sperm ejaculated at different times, not necessarily from the same male. The twins will be genetically different.

superfetation fertilisation of an ovum during a pregnancy. Extremely rare.

superior higher than, above.

superior longitudinal sinus the blood vessel which lies just under the skull bones in the mid-line and passes from front to back.

superior sagittal sinus one of six veins which drain blood from inside the skull into the jugular vein.

superior vena cava the major blood vessel which takes blood from the upper regions of the body back to the heart.

supination of the hand abnormality of the hand in which it turns upwards. Usually congenital.

supine lying flat on the back.

supine hypotensive syndrome a fall in the blood pressure which occurs when the pregnant woman lies on her back and she experiences a feeling of dizziness on rising. It is due to the gravid uterus compressing the vena cava and reducing venous return to the heart while the woman is supine.

supplement adding to, giving more than is normally available.

supplementary feed additional feed given after a breastfeed; also called a complementary feed.

support groups organisations whose members have common objectives or needs and that are willing to give assistance and encouragement to each other.

suppository medicine formed into a suitable shape which is inserted into the rectum where the drug is absorbed by the mucosa.

suppression to keep down against instinct, impulse or desire.

suppression of lactation prevention of milk secretion by natural methods such as binding or by drugs.

suppuration pus or discharge formation.

suprapubic the region above the pubis bones, found at the front of the abdomen.

suprapubic catheter a urinary catheter inserted through the skin just above the pubic bone following trauma or surgery to the pelvic floor.

surfactant a lipoprotein found in the lungs which keeps the alveoli inflated and reduces surface tension of the pulmonary fluids. It allows exchange of gases in the alveoli and aids the elasticity of pulmonary tissue. Preterm babies lack enough surfactant, making respiration laborious and potentially leading to the development of respiratory distress syndrome.

surgery the branch of medicine which attempts to treat conditions or improve function by means of cutting or operative procedures.

surrogate a person who fulfils the role of another.

surrogate mother a woman who conceives by natural or artificial means with the express intent of giving the child to another woman who is otherwise unable to have babies of her own.

survey a means of discovering information about the population by asking participants to complete a questionnaire or by observing their behaviour.

sustainable development goals (SDG) a set of 17 'Global Goals' with 169 targets. The SDGs were spearheaded by the United Nations and its 194 member states and were agreed in September 2015.

suture 1. a stitch used to close a wound.
2. membranous lines of indentation found on the fetal skull between two bones where calcification has not yet occurred. They allow moulding to occur in labour and close shortly after birth.

swaddling a method of wrapping a newborn baby that is thought to be comfortable and maintain warmth.

sweat test a method of diagnosing cystic fibrosis early in life. An area of skin is covered and sweating is induced. The sweat is collected and the salt levels analysed. Levels are raised three to six times above the normal in cystic fibrosis.

swimming reflex the innate ability of the infant to temporarily suspend respiration and make swimming movements when placed under water.

sympathetic showing a shared emotional understanding of another's problems and feelings.

sympathetic nervous system that part of the nervous system which prepares the body for 'fight or flight' by increasing the pulse, metabolic rate and blood pressure, dilating the pupils and slowing intestinal peristalsis.

symphysiotomy the cutting of the symphysis pubis to increase the pelvic diameters so that a large baby can pass through the pelvis (*see* Fig. 96); not performed in developed countries that have access to caesarean sections.

symphysis that part of the pelvic girdle made of strong cartilaginous tissue which lies between the pubic bones. It softens in pregnancy and increases the pelvic diameters.

symphysis fundal height measurement using a tape measure from the symphysis to the fundus. Used to monitor fetal growth during pregnancy.

symphysis pubis dysfunction (SPD) excessive softening of the cartilage with softening of the pubic bones and destabilisation of the joint.

symptom evidence of a condition or disease presented by the client.

sympus malformation of the feet in which extremities are fused or rotated.

syn-, sym- prefix meaning together.

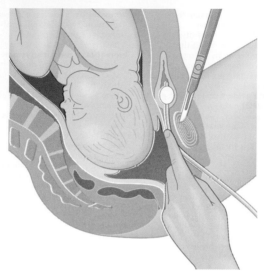

Figure 96
Symphysiotomy

synapse the junction where a nerve impulse moves to a different cell.

synclitism when the fetal head enters the pelvis straight, with both parietal bones level with the brim.

syncope loss of consciousness or fainting sometimes due to anaemia.

syncytiotrophoblast the multinucleated protoplasmic substance that surrounds the trophoblast.

syndactyly having webbing or skin layers between the fingers or toes.

syndrome a group of signs and symptoms which occur together in relation to a particular condition or disease.

synopsis a summary or a brief review, a précis.

synthesis 1. the binding together of substances not usually found together to form a compound. 2. the linking of previously analysed ideas or concepts to create new ideas, concepts or theories.

synthetic made artificially; not natural.

syphilis a sexually transmitted infection caused by the organism *Treponema pallidum*. It may cross the placental barrier in pregnancy and can cause abortion, stillbirth or congenital syphilis. In many countries, pregnant women are offered screening at booking. The infection is effectively treated with penicillin.

Système International d'Unités (International System of Units; SI units) an internationally agreed scale of measurement used in science, industry and pharmaceuticals. It uses metres, kilograms and seconds. (*See* Appendix 2.)

systemic referring to the whole of the body.

systole the contraction of the heart.

systolic relating to cardiac systole.

systolic murmur abnormal sound heard when the heart contracts.

systolic pressure the pressure exerted on the walls of the arteries when the heart contracts.

Tt

T-cell a special lymphocyte made in the bone marrow which matures in the thymus gland and is responsible for immunity and delayed hypersensitivity. The helper cell is a type of T-cell responsible for formation of antibodies by B-cells.

T4 cell helper cells which secrete interleukin-2 and stimulate production of natural killer cells, gamma interferon and the suppressor T8 cells. HIV can attack T4 cells resulting in the body's defences being severely damaged and enabling opportunistic infections to flourish.

tablet medicine prepared as a small solid pellet or disc which is usually taken orally and absorbed through the intestinal tract.

tabula rasa describes the mind of a child at birth as blank, clean or empty.

tachycardia fast heart rate.

tachypnoea fast respiratory rate.

tachysystole (uterine) uterine hyperstimulation, commonly defined as 5 or more contractions in a 10-minute period or contractions lasting longer than 90–120 seconds. Most commonly associated with the use of an oxytocin infusion.

tactile relating to touch, feeling a person or object with hands.

tail of Spence the upper outer segment of breast tissue found in the axilla.

talipes (club foot) the foot is bent inwards at birth (*see* Fig. 97). It may be caused by the position adopted in the uterus or be due to bone deformity.

talipomanus club hand.

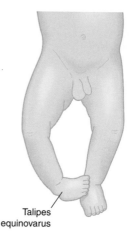

Talipes equinovarus

Figure 97
Talipes

talus the ankle bone.

tampon a wad of cotton wool or cloth with a thread or tape attachment; inserted into the vagina to absorb menstrual discharge.

tantrum a sudden display of anger usually caused by frustration; common in children aged about 2 years.

tarsus the seven bones of the ankle which allow the foot to rotate in all directions.

taurine a substance present in bile; it combines with cholic acid to make bile salts and enables conjugation of bilirubin.

Taussig-Bing syndrome an abnormal development of the heart in which there is transposition of the main vessels, accompanied by ventricular septal defect and ventricular hypertrophy.

Tay-Sachs disease an inherited neurodegenerative disorder of lipid metabolism caused by a deficiency of the enzyme hexosaminidase A. It is found among Ashkenazi Jews and can be detected antenatally by a maternal blood test. It causes progressive mental and physical decline and early death.

TBA (traditional birth attendant) definition applied by health organisations to a person, usually a woman, who accompanies a woman throughout labour and provides psychological support. The term is mainly used in low-resource countries. These women are often described as midwives within their own community and by other midwives who feel that midwifery expertise does not have to come from an institutionally based and nationally recognised program to be valid.

t.d.s. (LATIN *ter die sumendus*) instruction to give the prescribed medicine three times a day.

team midwifery a model of maternity care provided by a small team of midwives that focuses on continuity of care through pregnancy, labour and birth, and early parenting.

teething the eruption of teeth from the gums.

telangiectatic naevus a flat pink/purple area seen on the skin of the neonate where capillary dilation has occurred. Usually found on the back of the neck or head, eyelids, nose or upper lip.

telehealth the use of information and communications technologies (ICTs) to deliver health services and transmit health information over both long and short distances.

telemeter the recording and transmission of information by radio waves to a distal base station. The fetal heart can be monitored using this technology.

telemetry the recording of measurements that are then transmitted to receiving equipment remote to the point of collection. In maternity care, telemetry systems are used to monitor the fetal heart rate in women during labour so that they do not need to be physically connected to the monitor with wires.

temperament a personality type: happy, free and easy, melancholy, etc.

temperature the amount of heat in the body. Normal temperature is between 36°C and 37.5°C. Babies' temperatures can vary from 35.5°C to 37.5°C, the wide variation being due to an immature physiological mechanism.

temporal refers to the side part of the skull.

temporal bones the bones situated above the ear.

tenacious maintaining a firm hold; sticky, e.g. secretions such as mucus from the vagina.

tendon strong connective tissue which links a muscle to a bone.

TENS (transcutaneous electrical nerve stimulation) a method of pain relief used in labour. It is of uncertain physiology but may work by triggering the release of natural endorphins and enkephalins or by blocking (gate control theory) transmission of pain stimulus to the brain.

tension two forces exerting pressure in opposite directions.

tentorium cerebelli the fold of dura mater which extends horizontally inside the skull and separates the cerebral hemispheres from the cerebellum.

tepid slightly warm, up to 32°C.

ter in die (t.i.d.) (LATIN) used of medicine, meaning administer three times a day.

teras a malformed fetus or infant.

teratogen an agent that will cause fetal abnormalities if ingested or inhaled.

teratoma a congenital growth containing hair, nail or bone in an abnormal site.

term the natural end of pregnancy. Sometimes defined as 280 days or 40 weeks after the first day of the last normal menstrual period, or a period between 37 completed weeks and 42 completed weeks after the first day of the last normal menstrual period.

term infant a neonate born after 37 completed weeks' but before 43 weeks' gestation.

termination of pregnancy (TOP) a procedure intentionally performed to end a pregnancy usually before 14 weeks' gestation, although the timing can vary in different countries and contexts. Termination of pregnancy is not legal in all countries.

tertiary third stage, as in *tertiary syphilis*.

test procedure done to confirm or eliminate suggestion of possible disease. A *pregnancy test* is a laboratory procedure done to determine the presence of a pregnancy. *Glucose tolerance test* is a series of examinations of the blood after the person has been given a measured quantity of glucose orally (used to detect diabetes).

testes (SINGULAR testis; SYNONYM testicles) two glands located in the scrotum which produce spermatozoa and testosterone (*see* Fig. 98).

testicles *see* testes.

testicular relating to the testes.

testosterone male sex hormone responsible for male body characteristics and sex drive.

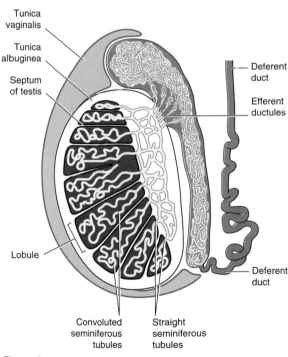

Tunica vaginalis

Tunica albuginea

Septum of testis

Lobule

Deferent duct

Efferent ductules

Deferent duct

Convoluted seminiferous tubules

Straight seminiferous tubules

Figure 98
Testes

tetanic related to tetanus, a painful tonic muscular spasm.

tetanus a disease caused by an anaerobic organism, *Clostridium tetani*, found naturally in soil. The organism causes spasm of muscles including those involved in respiration.

tetanus toxoid a preparation of detoxified tetanus toxin which will produce an immune response to *Clostridium tetani*.

tetany an abnormal condition caused by faulty calcium metabolism and associated with diminished function of the parathyroid glands. It is characterised by periodic painful muscular spasms and tremors.

tetracycline a broad-spectrum antibiotic contraindicated in pregnancy. It causes discolouration of the child's teeth and early degeneration of the first teeth.

tetradactyly congenital presence of only four digits on hands or feet.

tetralogy a collection of four things. As an example, in *Fallot's tetralogy* there are four congenital abnormalities affecting the heart: pulmonary stenosis, ventricular septal defect, dextroposition of the aorta and right ventricular hypertrophy.

tetraplegia paralysis of all four limbs.

thalamus a large ovoid mass in the posterior part of the forebrain. It relays sensory impulses to the cerebral cortex.

thalassaemia a haemoglobinopathy found in people of Mediterranean origin: the erythrocytes are abnormally small, pale and fragile. *Thalassaemia major*, the homozygous form, may present with severe haemolytic anaemia in childhood. *Thalassaemia minor* is the heterozygous form of the condition in which there is no clinical evidence of abnormality.

thalidomide a sedative and hypnotic drug formerly given to treat morning sickness but which caused severe limb abnormalities.

theca a capsule or enveloping sheath in which another structure is encased or protected.

theory an idea or a collection of arguable propositions used to explain an occurrence, situation or circumstance.

therapeutic relating to therapy; beneficial treatment.

therapeutic abortion termination of a pregnancy deemed necessary to preserve the health of the mother.

therapy treatment.

thermal refers to the production and maintenance of heat.

thermometer traditionally a small glass tube having a hollow vacuumed centre with a small amount of mercury which expands and rises according to the body temperature; now more commonly digital.

thermoneutral environment conditions designed so that the body temperature can be maintained with the least consumption of oxygen and energy.

thiamine vitamin B₁, part of the vitamin B complex required for neurological and cardiac functioning.

third stage of labour the stage of labour following the birth of the baby/babies until the placenta and membranes have been expelled and bleeding controlled, including management of haemorrhage if necessary.

thoracic referring to the thorax or chest cavity.

thorax the chest; that part of the body containing the lungs, heart, oesophagus and bronchi and enclosed by the diaphragm, vertebral column, ribs and sternum.

threatened abortion bleeding in early pregnancy without dilation of the cervix. The bleeding may stop and the pregnancy continue or the cervix may start to dilate making it an inevitable abortion.

threshold the level that must be reached before a certain reaction occurs.

thrill a tremor or vibration transmitted in fluid, felt by tapping the abdomen if polyhydramnios is present.

thrombectomy the surgical removal of a clot of blood from a vessel.

thrombin an enzyme liberated from shed blood that induces

clotting by converting the plasma protein fibrinogen into fibrin which forms a clot.

thrombocyte a blood platelet.

thrombocythaemia, thrombocytosis an abnormally large number of platelets in the blood.

thrombocytopenia an abnormally low number of platelets in the blood, occasionally seen in neonates.

thromboembolism part of a blood clot which has broken off and is circulating in the blood. When it reaches small vessels, it can cause a blockage.

thrombophlebitis inflammation of a vein with the formation of a clot; can occur during pregnancy as a result of the weight of the uterus on the vessels and sluggish venous return.

thromboplastin the substance liberated from damaged tissues which stimulates clot formation by acting on prothrombin.

thrombosis the formation of a thrombus or clot.

thrombus a clot caused by stasis of blood, usually in a vein.

thrush a fungal infection occurring in the vagina, mouth or sometimes between the toes. It is caused by *Candida albicans*. Neonates may contract it as a result of passing through an infected vagina or contact with the skin of the breast where there is poor hygiene.

thymus a gland that is responsible for coordinating

the development of the immune system and found in the front of the neck.

thyroid gland found anteriorly at the base of the neck, it straddles the trachea. This endocrine gland secretes thyroxin and triiodothyronine which control the metabolic rate. The Newborn Screening Test can detect underactivity of the gland in infants enabling early treatment which prevents cretinism.

thyrotoxic characterising the state that is produced by excessive quantities of thyroid hormone.

t.i.d. (LATIN *ter in die*) used of medicine, meaning administer three times a day.

tidal volume the volume of air inhaled and exhaled at each breath.

tingling prickling or vibrating sensation felt on the skin, usually in the path of a nerve.

tissue a mass of similar cells which act together to perform a specific function.

tissue fluid tiny amounts of fluid around the outside of each cell called extracellular fluid. Too much of this fluid is called oedema. It can occur towards the end of normal pregnancy around the ankles.

titre the amount of a substance administered according to the reaction in the body. Insulin is given in differing amounts according to the changing levels of glucose in the blood. A Syntocinon® infusion is titrated according to the contraction of the uterus, the dose being increased in labour until there are three contractions in 10 minutes or, where necessary, decreased to avoid over stimulation.

toco- a combining form meaning childbirth, derived from the Greek word *tokos*—birth.

tocograph a technique used to record the frequency and amplitude of contractions.

tocolytic a drug used to relax the muscles of the uterus and so stop contractions.

tocophobia fear of childbirth.

tocotransducer a piece of electronic equipment used to measure the pressure felt over the abdomen during a uterine contraction.

toddler a child between the age of 1 year and 3 years who is learning to walk and whose maturity and behaviour can be mapped according to a standard pattern.

TOLAC trial of labour after caesarean.

tolerance the body's ability to respond less aggressively to a substance due to continuous exposure.

tomograph radiological images of soft tissue made at various depths.

tone the amount of tension in a muscle.

tongue tie a congenital abnormality in which there is shortening of the frenulum— the fibrous tissue which anchors the tongue to the base of the mouth.

tonic contractions sustained uterine contractions, lasting longer than a minute thereby reducing placental perfusion to levels which may result in fetal hypoxia.

topical referring to direct application to a mucous membrane or the skin. Topical application comes in the form of a cream, paste, lotion or gel.

top-up additional administration of a substance, intended to elevate a declining level, for instance in epidural anaesthesia. The first 'top-up' injection of analgesic drug through the catheter into the epidural space is done by the anaesthetist. Subsequent top-ups may be administered by a midwife.

TORCH infection a group of infections (including toxoplasmosis, other [syphilis], rubella, cytomegalovirus and herpes) for which the neonate can be screened especially on admission to a special care unit.

torsion twisting; can occur to a tube, e.g. the fallopian tube, a hernia, the testes, the intestines or a cyst on the end of a stalk.

tort a wrong, breach of contract or act of negligence recognised in and by the law.

torticollis (SYNONYM cervical dystonia, spasmodic torticollis) a type of movement disorder in which the muscles controlling the neck cause sustained twisting or frequent jerking.

tourniquet a tight band of rubber or fabric applied to a limb to arrest haemorrhage or prevent emptying of a vein.

toxaemia toxins or poisons of some description in the blood.

toxic refers to a substance or gas which will cause severe deterioration in health.

toxic shock syndrome an acute bacterial infection caused by *Staphylococcus aureus* and characterised by fever, diarrhoea, erythematous rash and shock. It is thought to be associated with the use of tampons.

toxin a substance which can cause damage to health or congenital abnormalities if exposure should occur during pregnancy.

toxoid a toxin which has been treated with chemicals or heat to render it non-toxic but when introduced to the body can stimulate the production of antibodies.

toxoplasmosis a protozoal infection with influenza-like symptoms. If acquired in early pregnancy the infection can cross the placenta and infect the fetus causing miscarriage. Acquired in later pregnancy, it can cause multiple abnormalities in the baby.

trachea the windpipe, a cartilaginous cylinder which allows air to pass from the larynx to the bronchi.

trachelorrhaphy an operation to repair a torn cervix.

tracheo-oesophageal fistula a congenital abnormality in which there is a hole enabling communication between the trachea and the oesophagus. Food may pass into the lungs causing choking and air may pass into the stomach.

tracheostomy a surgical procedure to make an opening into the trachea (through the front of the neck).

traditional birth attendant see TBA.

trait characteristic feature of a disease or personality. A person with *sickle cell trait* has inherited one gene for sickle cell anaemia and can pass it on to his or her offspring.

tranexamic acid is in a class of medications called antifibrinolytics. It works to improve blood clotting and can be used for the management of post partum haemorrhage.

tranquilliser a drug which is used to calm an anxious person.

transcervical ligaments the bands of fibrous tissue which hold the cervix in position and are attached to the lateral walls of the pelvis.

transcutaneous bilirubinometer (TCB) an instrument which uses spectrophotometry to determine the levels of bilirubin present in the blood. This level is expressed as a measurement called TSB or total serum bilirubin.

transcutaneous electrical nerve stimulation see TENS.

transducer a machine which converts one form of energy into another capable of sending and receiving sound signals. When using ultrasound the transducer transforms electrical energy into vibrations of sound the frequency of which cannot be detected by the ear.

transferrin a serum globulin (protein) that binds and transports iron in the blood.

transfusion introduction of a substance directly into the bloodstream.

transient tachypnoea of the newborn a respiratory condition that appears soon after birth. The baby often shows chest retractions, expiratory grunting, or has cyanosis. Most babies recover with supportive management within 3 days.

transition a state of change; the period towards the end of the first stage of labour and the beginning of the second stage.

translocation the detachment of a part of one chromosome and attachment onto another.

transplacental across the placental barrier.

transport movement of material across or into cells.

transposition 1. a congenital abnormality in which one part of the body normally located on the right is found on the left and vice versa. 2. the shifting of genetic material from one chromosome to another. *Transposition of the great vessels* is a congenital heart anomaly in which the pulmonary artery arises from the left ventricle and the aorta from the right ventricle.

transudate fluid with very few particles which squeezes through cells or membranes.

transvaginal through the vagina.

transverse arrest interruption in the passage of the fetal head through the pelvis during labour. Rotation and descent are obstructed, usually by prominent ischial spines (*see* Fig. 99).

transverse lie the position of the fetal spine in relation to the mother's spine. The two are at right angles to each other. No presenting part can be identified.

transverse presentation the baby is lying across the uterus and the inlet of the pelvis.

transverse sinuses a pair of venous sinuses in the tentorium cerebelli under the skull.

trauma 1. sudden injury or damage to the body. 2. an incident which results in physical or emotional injury.

trauma-informed care a strengths-based approach, based on knowledge of the impact of trauma, aimed at ensuring environments and services are welcoming and engaging for service recipients and staff.

traumatic relating to or caused by trauma.

Trendelenburg position lying on the back with the body at an angle of 30 degrees and the head at the lowest point.

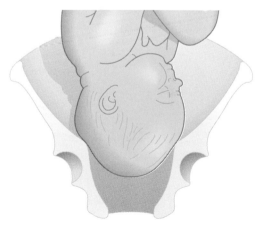

Figure 99
Transverse arrest

Treponema pallidum the spirochaete which causes syphilis.

trial of scar (trial of labour) historical term used to describe the desire to have a vaginal birth after a previous caesarean section (see NBAC, VBAC, TOLAC).

trichomoniasis, trichomonas vaginitis a common vaginal infection caused by a flagellate protozoan. Vaginal discharge may be watery, frothy, yellow/green.

trigone a triangular area at the base of the bladder between the ureters and the urethral openings (*see* Fig. 100). The area is not very elastic. As it lies against the anterior wall of the vagina the trigone may be damaged as the vagina distends in the second stage of labour.

trimester a period of 3 months. In pregnancy there are three trimesters, early, mid and last trimester.

tripartite three partitions or parts of a placenta each joined to the other by the cord.

triple test (SYNONYM triple screen) a genetic screening test often offered in the second trimester of pregnancy. This has now been replaced in many countries by nuchal translucency measurements or

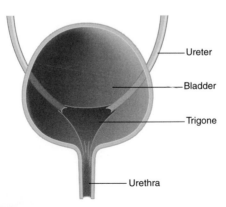

Figure 100
Trigone of bladder

non-invasive prenatal testing (*see* NIPT).

triplets three babies in the uterus or being born at the same time.

trisomy addition of a single chromosome to another pair, as in *trisomy 18* (Edwards' syndrome), *trisomy 21* (Down syndrome) and *trisomy 13* (Patau's syndrome).

trocar a sharp, pointed metal instrument fitted inside a cannula used for puncturing the body.

trochanter one of two bony prominences on the head of the femur bone.

trophoblast the outer layer of the blastocyst in embryonic life from which the placenta and chorionic membrane develop (*see* Fig. 101).

trophoblastic pertaining to the trophoblast, syncytiotrophoblast and cytotrophoblast.

true conjugate refers to the anterior–posterior diameter of the pelvic inlet, taken from

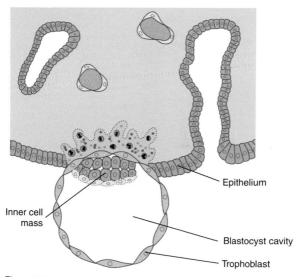

Epithelium

Inner cell mass

Blastocyst cavity

Trophoblast

Figure 101
Trophoblast

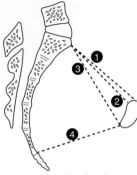

1. Anatomical/'true' conjugate
2. Obstetrical conjugate
3. Internal/diagonal conjugate
4. Obstetrical anterior–posterior of outlet

Figure 102
True conjugate

the sacral promontory to the centre of the upper surface of the symphysis pubis (*see* Fig. 102).

true labour uterine contractions which cause the cervix to dilate—as opposed to contractions which do not result in the birth of a baby.

tubal dermoid cyst a tumour containing embryonic tissue growing in an oviduct.

tubal insufflation dilation of the fallopian tubes. Carbon dioxide is pumped into the uterus and expected to pass through the fallopian tubes into the abdominal cavity. On X-ray the gas will be seen under the diaphragm, proving that the fallopian tubes are patent.

tubal ligation surgical tying and cutting of the fallopian tubes to prevent any meeting of ova and sperm.

tubal pregnancy development and implantation of the fertilised ovum in the fallopian tube.

tube feeding direct introduction of food into the stomach via the orogastric or nasogastric route.

tuberculosis a potentially fatal communicable infection caused by *Mycobacterium tuberculosis* that can affect almost any part of the body but is mainly an infection of the lungs.

tuberosity the thickened expanded portion of a bone. The *ischial tuberosity* is part of the ischial bone which is thick and upon which the body rests when in a sitting position.

tubo-ovarian abscess a capsule filled with infected material involving the ovary and fallopian tube.

tubo-ovarian cyst a fluid-filled sac involving the ovary and fallopian tube.

tubo-ovarian gestation an ectopic pregnancy which develops between the ovary and the fallopian tube.

tuboplasty surgical repair of the fallopian tube or restructuring to reverse a tubal ligation and restore fertility.

tubular necrosis death of cells in a tube, e.g. the nephrons, small tubules of the kidney. High blood pressure can cause the epithelial lining of the nephron to be damaged; this may block the nephron or cause release of toxins which will raise the blood pressure.

tubule microscopic tube in the nephron of the kidney.

tumour any abnormal growth in or on the body, arising from some particular tissue or cell type.

tunica an enveloping coat of fibrous connective membranes which covers an organ.

tunica albuginea a layer of connective tissue found below the germinal epithelium of the ovary.

tunnel a passage through solid material. The *carpal tunnel* is the passage between wrist bones through which the medial nerve and tendons pass to the hand. *Carpal tunnel syndrome* in pregnancy can occur when oedema causes pressure at this point on the medial nerve. An uncomfortable tingling sensation in the fingers may be felt.

Tuohy needle the blunt needle and cannula used to locate the epidural space around the spine.

Turner's syndrome a congenital abnormality in which there are 45 instead of 46 chromosomes. One of the sex chromosomes is absent so the child will appear female, have a vagina, uterus and fallopian tubes but the ovaries will not function.

twins two babies in the same uterus or being born at the same time. There are two types of twins: monozygotic (monovular) and dizygotic (binovular). Monozygotic twins are genetically identical individuals derived from a single fertilised egg. Dizygotic twins result when two different eggs undergo fertilisation by two different spermatozoa, not necessarily at the same time.

twin-to-twin transfusion transfer of blood from one fetus to the other resulting in one twin being polycythaemic, large and well nourished, while the other one is small, hypovolaemic and anaemic. Both babies are at risk of cardiac failure.

tympanic relating to or resembling a drum of the ear.

typhus an acute infectious illness transmitted to humans by rats and lice. Pyrexia, headache, rash and severe malaise will be present. The condition can be fatal.

typing the process of classifying blood tissues and other materials according to the characteristics they share.

Uu

ulcer a lesion on the skin or in the mucous membrane of the mouth or vagina, caused by trauma, infection or pressure on blood vessels. Healing is sometimes slow.

ulna the inner of the long bones in the forearm whose upper process forms the point of the elbow.

ultrasonic sound which cannot be heard with the ear, having in excess of 20 000 cycles per second. A transducer emits short pulses of high-frequency sound; these are bounced off structures within the body and the echoes collected and displayed on a screen.

ultrasonogram picture of an internal organ produced by ultrasound scanning.

ultrasonography the use of pulsed or continuous high frequency sound waves to observe the deep structures of the body.

ultrasound sound waves at a high frequency of over 20 000 kHz. It is used for examining the baby in utero, for dating, measuring growth and assessing for structural abnormalities.

ultraviolet light rays from the sun with extremely short wavelengths not visible to the human eye. They are grouped by types A, B, C and R according to wavelength and are able to penetrate the skin and cause burns. They are used in phototherapy units for treatment of neonates who are jaundiced. The light helps break down the bilirubin in the skin.

umbilical relating to the umbilicus.

umbilical catheterisation the passing of a fine catheter into the vein of the umbilicus and to the liver for purposes of feeding and assessing the condition of a sick neonate.

umbilical cord the cord containing (usually) two arteries and one vein which connects the baby to the placenta (*see* Fig. 103). Anomalies in the number of cord vessels may be indicative of kidney disease.

umbilical cord presentation the membranes are intact but the cord can be felt in front of the fetal head. (*See also* Fig. 22.)

umbilical cord prolapse the passage of the cord out of the uterus following rupture of the membranes. It may stay in the vagina or pass beyond the vulva in which case the cold air may cause the vessels to go into spasm stopping blood reaching the baby. Alternatively, the descent of the presenting part may compress the cord. Both

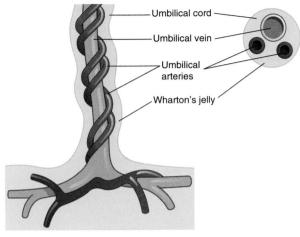

Figure 103
Umbilical cord

---

situations are obstetric emergencies usually requiring caesarean section.

umbilical hernia protrusion of the small intestines through a weakness in the muscular wall of the abdomen at the umbilicus. The swelling will become smaller as the child grows.

umbilical region area of the abdomen around the umbilicus; middle zone.

umbilical vein a vessel through which oxygenated blood passes from the placenta to the baby.

umbilicus the navel—the scar remaining after separation of the umbilical cord.

unconscious totally unaware of surroundings, unresponsive to stimuli.

unengaged head on abdominal examination the fetal head is palpated above the pelvic brim.

uni- prefix meaning one or single.

United Nations Children's Fund (UNICEF) a fund set up in 1946 by the United Nations to aid children in devastated areas of the world through provision of food, medical treatment, vaccinations, vitamins and education.

United Nations Population Fund (UNFPA) established by the United Nations with a focus on sexual and reproductive health services.

unicellular containing one cell only.

unilateral one side only.

uniovular one ovum (from which identical twins develop).

unisex 1. referring to only one gender. 2. having reproductive organs for one sex only. 3. clothing designed to be worn by both genders.

universal donor a person with blood group O Rh-negative who may give blood to any person without risk of a reaction.

universal precautions recommended standard of practice of all clinicians designed to prevent transmission of infectious diseases including HIV and hepatitis. It includes the wearing of protective layers of clothing and cleaning procedures including hand washing.

universal recipient a person with blood group AB Rh-positive who may receive blood from any person without a reaction.

unstable lie refers to the continuing changing lie of the fetus in utero. It cannot be predicted what the lie will be when labour starts. There is a risk of cord prolapse.

upper respiratory tract infection (URTI) includes colds, tonsillitis, pharyngitis, rhinitis and laryngitis.

urachus a canal present in a fetus that connects the bladder with the allantois via the navel. It mostly disappears in the neonatal period.

uraemia term implying excessive uric acid in the blood. This is a pathophysiological state resulting from renal failure. There is acidosis, disturbance in electrolyte balance, sodium and water retention, oedema and hyperkalaemia.

uranoschisis cleft palate.

uranostaphyloplasty the surgical repair of a cleft palate.

urate salts derived from uric acid, found in blood. They may be deposited in joints and referred to as gout.

urea the excreted product of protein metabolism. It is filtered out of the blood by the kidneys and passed down to the bladder for voiding at a suitable time. Blood urea level is normally 2.5–5.8 mmol/L.

ureter tube which passes from the kidneys to the bladder and carries urine. The effect of high levels of progesterone in pregnancy cause dilation and stasis of urine in the ureters with an increased risk of infection.

ureteric referring to the ureters.

ureteritis inflammation or infection in the ureter.

urethra tube from the bladder to the external orifice through which urine is discharged. It is 20 cm long in the male and 3.5 cm in the female. It can be stretched or bruised during childbirth especially in association with forceps delivery. This can lead to urinary retention and overflow incontinence.

urethral referring to the urethra.

urethral sphincter the voluntary muscle at the neck of the bladder which relaxes during urination.

urethrocele herniation of the wall of the urethra so that it protrudes into the vagina.

urethrocystitis inflammation of the urethra and bladder.

uric referring to urine.

uric acid the product of protein metabolism, found in the blood (0.13–0.42 mmol/L) and urine (less than 1 g/day).

urinalysis physical, biochemical and microscopic examination of the urine to detect abnormalities. During pregnancy urine is examined for glucose to detect intolerance or diabetes, protein to detect pre-eclampsia or infection, ketones to detect dehydration or fat metabolism and blood to detect infection or kidney damage.

urinary related to urine.

urinary frequency the desire to void urine very often.

urinary ileostomy the surgical construction of a passage from the bladder to the ilium, which is then used as a urinary reservoir.

urinary incontinence involuntary passage of urine; the inability to control the bladder sphincter leading to leakage of urine.

urinary retention the state where the bladder cannot be emptied despite the desire to do so. Can occur following forceps delivery, epidural anaesthesia, caesarean section, cases of incarcerated gravid uterus and anterior vaginal wall laceration. The bladder will be palpable abdominally.

urinary tract infection (UTI) bacterial growth in the urinary tract. The presence of pus turns the urine cloudy. Potential complications of UTI include kidney damage and possibly preterm labour.

urination the act of passing urine.

urine the clear, straw-coloured fluid secreted by the kidneys as a result of filtering impurities out of the blood.

urinometer a glass cylinder into which urine is collected and a float deposited, used to measure the specific gravity of the urine.

urobilinogen a colourless compound formed in the intestines after the breakdown of bilirubin and present in urine.

urodynamics the dynamics of the propulsion and flow of urine in the urinary tract.

URTI *see* upper respiratory tract infection.

urticaria characteristic reaction in which the skin is raised and itchy.

uterine referring to the uterus.

uterine bruit the sound heard with a stethoscope as blood pulsates through the arteries of the uterus.

uterine prolapse descent of the uterus from its normal location in the vagina due to weakened pelvic floor muscles.

uterine souffle a soft blowing sound heard as the blood passes through the vessels of the placenta.

uterine tetany prolonged uterine contractions.

uteroplacental referring to the junction where the placenta meets the inner lining of the uterus.

uterosacral referring to the uterus and the sacrum.

uterosacral ligament a thick fibrous band connecting the cervix to the sacrum and offering support to the uterus.

uterosalpingography radiological examination of the uterus and fallopian tubes. Radioactive dye is introduced into the uterus and left to track into the fallopian/uterine tube and X-rays are taken to detect defects.

uterotomy (SYNONYM hysterotomy) cutting into the uterus.

uterovesical referring to the uterus and the bladder.

uterovesical pouch the fold of peritoneum between the bladder and the uterus.

uterus the womb, the organ which receives and grows the fertilised ovum during development of the fetus and actively participates in its expulsion as part of the birthing process (*see* Fig. 104).

uterus bicornis (bicornate uterus) a uterus which divides in two at the upper pole but is fused at the lower pole.

UTI *see* urinary tract infection.

utilitarianism an ethical concept which states that all action should be guided by the desire to bring about the greatest happiness for the greatest number of people.

uvula soft, fleshy pendant hanging from the edge of the soft palate at the back of the mouth.

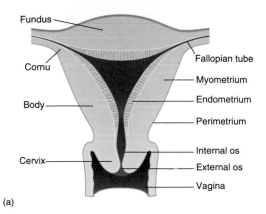

Fundus

Cornu

Body

Cervix

Fallopian tube

Myometrium

Endometrium

Perimetrium

Internal os

External os

Vagina

(a)

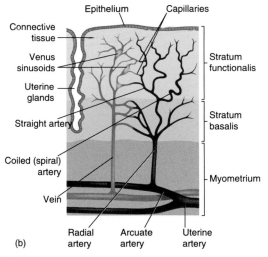

Epithelium

Capillaries

Connective tissue

Venus sinusoids

Uterine glands

Straight artery

Coiled (spiral) artery

Vein

Stratum functionalis

Stratum basalis

Myometrium

Radial artery

Arcuate artery

Uterine artery

(b)

Figure 104
Uterus

vaccinate to inoculate or introduce a vaccine into the body.

vaccination an injection of attenuated (weakened) microorganisms, bacteria or viruses which may induce immunity or reduce the effects of a disease.

vaccine the suspension of attenuated or killed microorganisms which is administered during vaccination.

vacuum aspiration
1. withdrawal of substances using negative pressure.
2. termination of an early pregnancy by suction out of the uterus through the cervix.

vacuum extraction *see* ventouse extraction.

vagal referring to the vagus nerve.

vagina hollow tube 10 cm long extending from the vulva to the cervix. The lining of squamous epithelium is in folds or rugae which will stretch easily.

vaginal referring to the vagina.

vaginal atrophy postmenopausal condition occurring where oestrogen levels are lowered.

vaginal bleeding may be from a local ulceration of the vagina or from the uterus in pregnancy which is called an antepartum haemorrhage (APH) or threatened abortion, depending on gestation.

vaginal cyst abnormal closed sac or pouch, filled with fluid or connective tissue.

vaginal delivery birth of a fetus through the vagina. More commonly expressed as vaginal birth.

vaginal discharge an emission or secretion that may be clear or pearly white, containing endocervical cells. If offensive or green it can indicate infection.

vaginal examination (VE) examination per vaginam.

vaginal fornix a recess in the upper part of the vaginal canal caused by protrusion of the cervix.

vaginal hysterectomy removal of the uterus through an incision in the vagina.

vaginal jelly common term applied to a contraceptive product containing a spermicide. Used in conjunction with a contraceptive diaphragm or cervical cap to occlude the cervix and prevent pregnancy occurring.

vaginal lubricant an ointment or cream used to reduce friction in the vagina during intercourse or vaginal examination.

vaginal septum a fold of tissue dividing the length of the vagina. A congenital abnormality caused by incomplete development of the genitalia in embryonic life.

vaginal speculum an instrument with two curved blades which can be inserted into the vagina and opened to allow for inspection of the walls and cervix.

vaginismus painful spasm of vaginal muscles.

vaginitis inflammation of the vagina. May be due to a fungus (*Candida albicans*) or to a flagellate protozoan (*Trichomonas vaginalis*), both of which cause a discharge and itching.

vagus the 10th cranial nerve which supplies and stimulates the lungs, heart, liver and stomach.

valgus a turning away from the mid-line of the body, e.g. *talipes valgus*.

validity the extent to which a test measurement or other device measures what it is intended to measure.

Valsalva manoeuvre 1. a procedure originally created to aid the expulsion of ear wax whereby increased intrathoracic pressure is achieved by closing the glottis and forcing expiration. Has been used during the second stage of labour to cause pressure to increase in the abdomen thereby aiding the bearing-down efforts of the mother to deliver the baby. The practice is no longer encouraged as it is thought to contribute to fetal distress. 2. performed spontaneously by infants with respiratory distress syndrome to maintain a positive pressure in the thorax during expiration. A grunt results.

value 1. a belief about the worth of a given idea or behaviour. 2. a quantitative measurement of the activity or concentration of specific substances found in healthy tissue, blood, secretions, etc.

valve a natural or artificial structure present in a vessel which prevents backward flow of its contents.

vaping the process by which vapour from an e-cigarette is inhaled (*see also* e-cigarette).

variable a factor in an experiment or quantitative element that differs in values under changing conditions, e.g. the pulse at rest, during light exercise or during maximal exertion.

variance a numerical representation of the dispersion of data around the mean in a sample of results of research.

varicella a herpes-like viral infection. Causes chickenpox or shingles (herpes zoster).

varicose veins distended, bulging, dilated veins. The valves do not close efficiently allowing backflow of blood. In pregnancy the condition occurs under the influence of the hormone progesterone. Varicose veins may appear on the legs, vulva (vulvar varicosities) and around the anus (haemorrhoids).

variola smallpox.

varix an enlarged vein or a distended twisted lymphatic vessel.

vas a tube or vessel.

vas deferens the tube which carries spermatozoa from the testis to the male urethra.

vasa praevia the vessels from a velamentous insertion of the umbilical cord which run into the membranes, through to the placenta, and pass between the presenting part and the cervical opening. When the membranes rupture there is a risk that the vessels will rupture causing exsanguination, hypoxia, brain damage or death of the fetus.

vascular referring to blood vessels, usually small ones.

vascularity the amount of blood vessels in a given area or organ.

vasectomy dissection and excision of part of the vas deferens, to prevent passage of spermatozoa (*see* Fig. 105). The man is usually sterile after 3 months.

vasoconstrictor a drug, hormone or enzyme which causes narrowing of the lumen of blood vessels. It will affect blood pressure and the distribution of blood throughout the body.

vasodepressor an agent causing reduction of peripheral resistance to blood flow and resulting in lowering of blood pressure.

vasodilator a drug, hormone or enzyme which causes dilation of blood vessels by making smooth muscles of the vessels relax.

vasomotor referring to the nerves which control the contraction and relaxation of muscles of the blood vessels.

vasopressin a hormone produced by the posterior lobe of the pituitary gland and which acts on the kidneys to control water balance in the body. It has a marked antidiuretic property.

vasopressor usually a drug or hormone which stimulates contraction of the smooth muscle of vessels.

vault 1. a dome-shaped structure. 2. the top part of the fetal skull which contains the cerebral hemispheres. Made up of two parietal bones, two frontal bones and the occiput. They are divided by membranes and fontanelles which allow overlapping (moulding) during birth (*see* Fig. 106).

VBAC vaginal birth after caesarean.

VDRL (Venereal Disease Research Laboratory) refers to a test which is done to detect syphilis.

vegan a person who does not eat or use any products of animal origin, that is, meat, fish, dairy, eggs, leather, honey. Vegan women may also decline the routine use of pharmaceutical drugs derived from animal products, e.g. oxytocics, prostaglandins.

vegetarian a person who does not eat meat, fish or foods

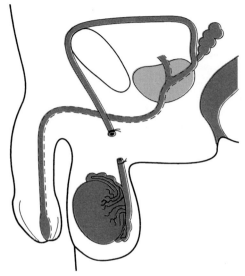

Figure 105
Vasectomy

made from the bodies of
animals; a *lacto-ovo
vegetarian* will eat dairy
products and eggs; *complete
vegetarian* is another term for
vegan.
vein a vessel in the circulatory
system which carries blood
towards the heart.
vein of Galen the large
cerebral vein that drains
blood from the mid-brain.
velamentous veil-like.
**velamentous insertion of the
cord** the cord is anchored in

the membranes and the
vessels divide before reaching
the placenta (*see* Fig. 107).
vena cava two major veins
running the length of the
spine which return blood to
the right upper chamber of
the heart. The abdominal
section can be compressed by
the uterus when the pregnant
woman lies on her back.
Venous return to the heart
will be inhibited causing
pooling of blood in the
abdominal cavity and reduced

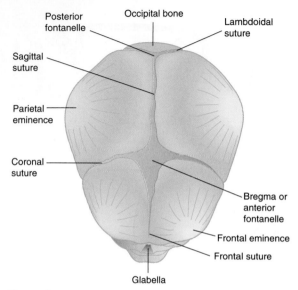

Figure 106
Vault of fetal skull

supply to the head. Dizziness, low blood pressure and fainting may result.

venepuncture perforation of a vein to obtain a specimen of blood for diagnostic testing.

venereal referring to sexual intercourse. *Venereal disease* is an infection transmitted from one person to another by sexual intercourse.

venesection opening of the vein to take blood or introduce drugs.

venous stasis pooling or cessation in the flow of blood in a vein.

venous thrombosis formation of a blood clot in a vein which obstructs the blood flow through the vessel.

ventilation introduction of air into a room, or into the lungs by artificial means.

ventilator an apparatus used to force air mixed with oxygen into the lungs via an endotracheal tube using

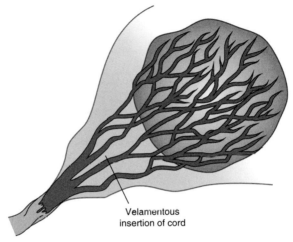

Velamentous
insertion of cord

Figure 107
Velamentous insertion of the cord
Illustration by Alan Laver

continuous or intermittent pressure.

ventouse extraction (vacuum extraction) the application of a cap to the fetal head when completion of the second stage of labour is delayed. The cap is attached to a machine or part of an apparatus which creates negative pressure. Traction can be applied which, with maternal efforts, may achieve birth. This aids the mother's efforts to deliver the baby without recourse to application of forceps.

ventricle a small cavity such as the lower chambers of the heart or the cavities in the brain filled with cerebrospinal fluid.

ventricular septal defect refers to a congenital abnormality of the heart. The wall dividing the right and left side of the heart is patent allowing blood from one side of the heart to flow to the other, bypassing the lungs.

ventrosuspension surgical procedure in which the abdomen is opened and the round ligaments supporting the uterus are shortened to change the uterus from being retroverted to anteverted.

venule a tiny vein.

vernix caseosa a greasy substance secreted from the sebaceous glands. It covers the fetus in utero and falls off into the liquor at term.

verruca contagious skin condition caused by a virus.

version turning of the fetal position in utero. Cephalic version is turning to make the head present over the internal os. In external cephalic version (ECV) the fetus is manipulated through the abdominal wall until it is a cephalic presentation. Podalic version is turning the fetus to a breech position from an oblique lie or following delivery of a first twin. In internal version the operator's hand is introduced into the uterus and a second twin is turned from a transverse lie in order to achieve a vaginal birth.

vertebrae (SINGULAR vertebra) the irregular-shaped bones which form the spine and through the middle of which passes the spinal cord.

vertebral canal hollow channel in the vertebrae through which the spinal cord passes.

vertebral column the structure composed of 33 vertebrae resting one on top of another and divided by cartilage which encases the spinal cord, maintains rigidity and provides support to the upper body.

vertex the top of the fetal head bounded by the anterior and posterior fontanelles and the parietal eminences.

vertigo a sensation described as dizziness.

vesica the urinary bladder.

vesical referring to the urinary bladder or other fluid-filled sac.

vesical fistula an abnormal opening into the urinary bladder.

vesical sphincter the circular muscle which closes the bladder.

vesicle a blister or small sac usually containing fluid.

vesicouterine referring to the bladder and the uterus.

vesicovaginal referring to the bladder and vagina.

vesicular referring to or containing vesicles.

vestibule 1. entrance or passageway. 2. part of the vulva found between the labia minora.

vestige the remnants of a structure from fetal life.

viable capable of survival.

vicarious liability describes an agreement where an employer has responsibility for the actions carried out in the course of the employee's work.

villi fine, hair-like processes which project from skin or a mucous surface. Found in the lungs, intestines and placenta. *Chorionic villi* are processes around the trophoblast which grow into the maternal blood vessels.

viraemia viral infection of the blood.

viral referring to a virus.

viral infection occurring where a virus enters the body and attaches itself to a susceptible cell which absorbs the virus. The virus matures inside the cell using its own genetic information. It replicates itself in the parasitised cell. It will then appear outside the cell and seek new cells to parasitise.

viral load test a measurement of the amount of the human immunodeficiency virus in the blood.

virgin 1. a person who has never had sexual intercourse. 2. pure, uncontaminated.

virus very small microorganism which can only grow within another cell. Viruses can cross the placental barrier and cause congenital abnormalities in the first trimester.

viscera internal organs enclosed within a body cavity.

visceral cavity the abdominal cavity; the cavity of any organ, e.g. the stomach.

viscosity the resistance exhibited by a fluid as it flows over a surface.

viscous sticky, as thick mucus.

visual analogue scale (VAS) a method of quantifying feelings, e.g. pain. A line is drawn, one end representing no pain sensation the other severe pain. The person is asked to plot the strength of his or her pain on the line. This may be used again to detect changes in the level of pain.

visual disturbance impairment of visual acuity. May be due to optic or cerebral oedema and may indicate the presence of pre-eclampsia or impending convulsion.

vital 1. very important. 2. relating to life.

vital signs temperature, pulse, respiratory rate, blood pressure, level of consciousness and responsiveness.

vital statistics record of births and deaths including causative factors in the population maintained by the births, deaths and marriage registries.

vitamin essential food substances, minute amounts of which are necessary for health. Early classification divided them into groups from A to V. Deficiency of vitamins causes an array of conditions depending on which one is absent from the diet.

vitamin K deficiency disorder a lack of vitamin K in infants may result in life-threatening bleeding within the skull (intracranial haemorrhage).

vitellin a protein containing lecithin found in egg yolk.

vitelline artery the vessels which circulate blood through the yolk sac to and from the embryo.

vitellus the yolk of an ovum.

viviparous classification of species that give birth to live offspring.

void to empty, usually the bladder.

voluntary an action or thought involving conscious decision.

volvulus twisting, usually of the intestines, causing an obstruction or strangulation.

vomiting forceful expulsion of the contents of the stomach; sign of a pathological process. *Projectile vomiting* is very forceful vomiting usually caused by pyloric stenosis. *Vomiting in the newborn* may be due to overfeeding, air or mucus in the stomach. *Vomiting in early pregnancy* is commonly called morning sickness; more usually the woman is nauseous due to the presence of unfamiliar hormones in quantity in the brain. *Severe vomiting in pregnancy* (hyperemesis gravidarum) can result in dehydration and electrolyte imbalance. *Vomiting in late pregnancy* may be due to impending eclampsia, gastroenteritis or the onset of labour.

vomitus the material which comes up from the stomach.

vulsellum a type of forceps.

vulva external part of the female genital organs.

vulvectomy cutting away of the vulva.

vulvitis inflammation of the vulva.

warfarin an oral anticoagulant drug which will cross the placental barrier. Only given between 16 and 36 weeks' gestation if clinically indicated.

wart a virus which invades the skin only causing a roughened elevation. *Genital warts* are found on the vulva, perineum and anal regions. They can be treated topically.

Wassermann reaction specific antibody test for syphilis.

water birth birthing of the baby in water.

water intoxication excess water in the body to the extent that bodily functions are impaired.

waterborne protein, salt or microorganism which moves about in water.

weaning changing the diet in an infant. There is a gradual change from milk to semi-solid foods and then solid foods slowly over several months.

webbed connected by a fold of membrane or skin. These are more usually found between the toes and fingers.

wedge resection surgical removal of a wedge-shaped part of an organ, usually the ovary or cervix.

wellbeing individual sense of contentment with state of health.

Wernicke's encephalopathy acute haemorrhagic encephalitis associated with severe hyperemesis gravidarum.

Wertheim's operation hysterectomy which is combined with removal of the ovaries, fallopian tubes, upper third of the vagina, perimetrium and clearance of pelvic lymph nodes. Used to treat cancer of the cervix.

wet nurse a woman who breastfeeds babies who are not her own.

Wharton's jelly the clear jelly-like substance surrounding the vessels of the umbilical cord.

whey the fluid part of milk which can be separated from the solid part (curds).

white asphyxia a term formerly used to refer to a baby born with a low Apgar score who appeared 'white' at birth. *See* asphyxia.

white blood cell (WBC) leucocytes found in the blood. Their function is to ingest foreign bodies and microorganisms.

white coat hypertension (WCH) people with normal blood pressure in their usual environment find it is increased when measured by a clinician.

white matter white substance composed of myelinated nerve fibres, responsible for transmission of impulses up the spinal cord and across the brain.

WHO International Code of Marketing of Breast Milk Substitutes a campaign started in conjunction with UNICEF to safeguard breastfeeding practice and regulate the advertising of breast-milk substitutes by companies in developing countries. The code prevents direct advertising, free distribution of samples, special offers and discounts to mothers and professionals.

whole blood donated blood is transfused without the removal of any components.

whooping cough *see* pertussis.

Wilson–Mikity syndrome a condition occurring in babies who have needed to be ventilated for a period of time; the lung tissue loses its elasticity.

withdrawal bleeding blood loss from the uterus occurring after the cessation of oestrogen and progesterone preparations, as happens with each course of oral contraceptive pills.

withdrawal method practice during intercourse in which the penis is removed from the vagina just before ejaculation.

withdrawal symptoms unpleasant, possibly damaging, symptoms which occur after cessation of a drug taken regularly for a long period of time.

wolffian bodies two small organs in the embryo, which are the primitive kidneys.

woman-centred care an important concept in midwifery practice that highlights the importance of basing care on the needs expectations and aspirations of an individual woman, rather than an institution or profession. The definition includes the need to recognise the woman's right to self-determination, includes the needs of the baby, her family and significant others and follows the woman across the interface between institutions and the community.

womb uterus.

Woolwich shell a plastic domed appliance with a flat base containing a hole. Used to encourage retraction of flat nipples. The nipple is inserted into the hole and the appliance is worn inside the brassiere.

woods screw manoeuvre rotational manoeuvres designed to internally rotate the baby's shoulders using the accoucher's fingers so that the shoulders can come under the maternal symphysis.

World Health Organization (WHO) special agency set up by the United Nations Council which is concerned with international health. It funds research and development, and supports educational and local initiatives to improve environmental health. It initiated the Safe Motherhood campaign to improve maternal mortality in underdeveloped countries.

wound injury caused to the skin and underlying tissues by surgery, trauma or puncture.

wound healing process whereby integrity and function are restored to an injured part.

Wrigley's forceps obstetric forceps used to grip the fetal head. Traction is applied to effect birth of the baby when the second stage of labour is delayed. The head needs to be low in the pelvic cavity for a 'lift out'. They are also used during caesarean section or to control the aftercoming head in an obstetrically managed breech birth.

Xx

X chromosome one of two chromosomes that determine the gender of a cell. A cell with XX chromosomes will be female and a cell with XY chromosomes will be male.

xanthoderma skin with a yellow tinge, as in jaundice.

xenogenesis the changing of genes as they are passed down several generations to produce different traits.

xeroderma skin that is dry and rough.

xeromammogram a type of X-ray using metal plates instead of films for examining the breast.

xiphoid process a small piece of cartilage at the end of the sternum against which the height of the uterine fundus is measured during pregnancy.

X-linked refers to a disease acquired by recessive inheritance in which the defect is located on the X chromosome. The female will carry the condition without being affected and will pass it on to her male children who will be affected.

X-linked dominant inheritance passing on of a characteristic expressed whenever the gene is present on the X chromosome.

X-linked inheritance the passing on of traits on the X chromosome. These traits are maternally derived and will not be passed on by males to their sons but their daughters will be carriers and will pass it on to the next generation.

X-linked recessive inheritance a pattern of inheritance in which the females carry the trait and only the males show symptoms.

XO denotes a condition called Turner's syndrome in which only one chromosome (X) is present in each cell.

X-ray pelvimetry radiological picture of the pelvis which can be measured to determine the dimensions. Rarely carried out in current practice.

X-rays electromagnetic waves which can pass through many substances such as skin, muscle and paper but are absorbed by lead, bone and platinum. When a part of the skeleton is exposed to X-ray, images can be made of the bones and diseases including fractures detected.

XYY syndrome a condition in which the male has an extra Y chromosome making 47 in each cell instead of 46. The male is often aggressive and tall, and displays antisocial behaviour.

Yy

Y chromosome the sex chromosome indicative of a male.

yaws a disease found in the tropics that resembles syphilis and is caused by *Treponema* but which is not a venereal disease. Tests for syphilis will be positive.

yeast a specific fungus which causes fruit juices and malt to ferment producing alcohol.

Thrush is a yeast-type infection caused by *Candida albicans*.

yolk sac a structure that develops in the inner cell mass and expands into a vesicle with a thick stalk that becomes the embryonic gut (*see* Fig. 108). It supplies the nourishment for the developing embryo and disappears by the 7th week of gestation.

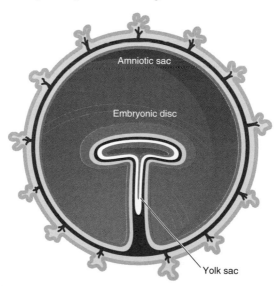

Figure 108
Yolk sac

Zz

zero (0) the symbol meaning 'o'—nought or nothing. It is also the point on a centigrade thermometer at which temperature measurement begins, water turns to ice or above which ice melts.

zika an infection caused by an arbovirus of the *Flaviviridae* family that is carried by mosquitos. It does not usually cause symptoms but has been associated with congenital abnormalities when pregnant women become infected.

zinc an element essential in the diet for making enzymes. Deficiency can cause growth restriction in children, low sperm counts in men and slow wound healing.

zona fasciculata the middle part of the adrenal cortex which produces glucocorticoids and sex hormones.

zona pellucida the thick transparent secretory layer surrounding the ovum. A sperm's head contains an enzyme which digests this layer allowing penetration and fertilisation.

zygogenesis joining to form a single unit; the formation of the zygote after fertilisation.

zygote the fertilised ovum before it starts to divide.

zygote intrafallopian transfer (ZIFT) infertility treatment. Introduction of the fertilised ovum (prior to segmentation) into the fallopian tube.

Appendix 1

Conversion charts

Measurements, equivalents and conversions (SI or metric and imperial)

Length
1 kilometre (km)	= 1000 metres (m)
1 metre (m)	= 100 centimetres (cm) or 1000 millimetres (mm)
1 centimetre (cm)	= 10 millimetres (mm)
1 millimetre (mm)	= 1000 micrometres (μm)
1 micrometre (μm)	= 1000 nanometres (nm)

Volume
1 litre (L)	= 1000 millilitres (mL)
1 millilitre (mL)	= 1000 microlitres (μL)

Note: The millilitre (mL) and the cubic centimetre (cm^3) are usually treated as being the same.

Conversions
1 litre (L)	= 1.76 pints (pt) (Australia, NZ, UK)
1 litre (L)	= 2.20 pints (pt) (US)
568.25 millilitres (mL)	= 1 pint (pt) (Australia, NZ, UK)
454.55 millilitres (mL)	= 1 pint (pt) (US)
28.4 millilitres (mL)	= 1 fluid ounce (fl oz)

Weight or mass
1 kilogram (kg)	= 1000 grams (g)
1 gram (g)	= 1000 milligrams (mg)
1 milligram (mg)	= 1000 micrograms (μg)
1 microgram (μg)	= 1000 nanograms (ng)

Note: To avoid any confusion with milligram (mg) the word microgram (μg) should be written in full on prescriptions.

Conversions
1 kilogram (kg)	= 2.204 pounds (lb)
1 gram (g)	= 0.0353 ounce (oz)
453.59 grams (g)	= 1 pound (lb)
28.34 grams (g)	= 1 ounce (oz)

Temperature conversions
To convert centigrade to Fahrenheit:
multiply by 9, divide by 5, and add 32 to the result
e.g. 36°C to Fahrenheit:
$36 \times 9 = 324 \div 5 = 64.8 + 32 = 96.8°F$
therefore 36°C = 96.8°F
To convert Fahrenheit to centigrade:
subtract 32, multiply by 5, and divide by 9
e.g. 104°F to centigrade:
$104 - 32 = 72 \times 5 = 360 \div 9 = 40°C$
therefore 104°F = 40°C

Appendix 2

SI units

Base units

Quantity	Base unit and symbol
Length	metre (m)
Mass	kilogram (kg)
Time	second (s)
Amount of substance	mole (mol)
Electric current	ampere (A)
Thermodynamic temperature	kelvin (K)
Luminous intensity	candela (cd)

Quantity	Derived unit and symbol
Work, energy, quantity of heat	joule (J)
Pressure	pascal (Pa)
Force	newton (N)
Frequency	hertz (Hz)
Power	watt (W)
Electrical potential, electromotive force, potential difference	volt (v)
Absorbed dose of radiation	gray (Gy)
Radioactivity	becquerel (Bq)
Dose equivalent	sievert (Sv)

Multiplication factor	Prefix	Symbol
10^{12}	tera	T
10^{9}	giga	G
10^{6}	mega	M
10^{3}	kilo	k
10^{2}	hecto	h
10^{1}	deca	da
10^{-1}	deci	d
10^{-2}	centi	c
10^{-3}	milli	m
10^{-6}	micro	μ
10^{-9}	nano	n
10^{-12}	pico	p
10^{-15}	femto	f
10^{-18}	atto	a

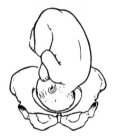

Figure A3.1
Left occipitoanterior

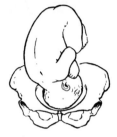

Figure A3.2
Right occipitoanterior

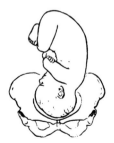

Figure A3.3
Left occipitolateral

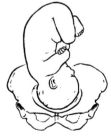

Figure A3.4
Right occipitolateral

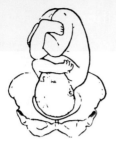

Figure A3.5
Left occipitoposterior

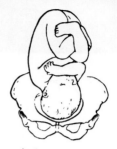

Figure A3.6
Right occipitoposterior

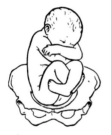

Figure A3.7
Right sacroposterior

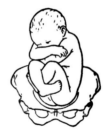

Figure A3.8
Left sacroposterior

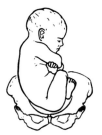

Figure A3.9
Right sacrolateral

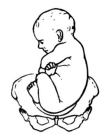

Figure A3.10
Left sacrolateral

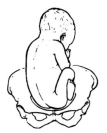

Figure A3.11
Right sacroanterior

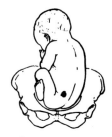

Figure A3.12
Left sacroanterior

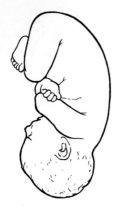

Figure A3.13
Vertex (well-flexed head)

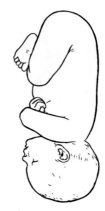

Figure A3.14
Vertex (deflexed head)

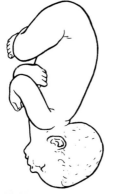

Figure A3.15
Brow (partially extended head)

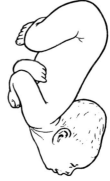

Figure A3.16
Face (fully extended head)

Appendix 4

Classification of perineal tears

Degree	Trauma
First	Injury to the perineal skin and/or vaginal mucosa
Second	Injury to the perineum involving perineal muscles but not involving the anal sphincter
Third	Injury to perineum involving the anal sphincter complex: Grade 3a: less than 50% of external anal sphincter (EAS) thickness torn Grade 3b: more than 50% of EAS thickness torn Grade 3c: both EAS and internal anal sphincter (IAS) torn
Fourth	Injury to perineum involving the anal sphincter complex (EAS and IAS) and ano-rectal mucosa

Source: Royal College of Obstetricians and Gynaecologists (RCOG). *The management of third- and fourth-degree perineal tears. Green-top guideline no. 29.* London: ROCH; 2015.

Female genital mutilation classification system[1]

The extent of female genital mutilation (FGM) can be classified according to the degree of injury/incision.

Type I	Partial or total removal of the clitoris and/or the prepuce (clitoridectomy). When it is important to distinguish between the major variations of Type I mutilation, the following subdivisions are commonly used: • Type Ia, removal of the clitoral hood or prepuce only; • Type Ib, removal of the clitoris with the prepuce.
Type II	Partial or total removal of the clitoris and the labia minora, with or without excision of the labia majora (excision). When it is important to distinguish between the major variations that have been documented, the following subdivisions are commonly used: • Type IIa, removal of the labia minora only; • Type IIb, partial or total removal of the clitoris and the labia minora; • Type IIc, partial or total removal of the clitoris, the labia minora and the labia majora.
Type III	Narrowing of the vaginal orifice with creation of a covering seal by cutting and appositioning the labia minora and/or the labia majora, with or without excision of the clitoris (infibulation). When it is important to distinguish between variations in infibulations, the following subdivisions are commonly used: • Type IIIa, removal and apposition of the labia minora; • Type IIIb, removal and apposition of the labia majora.
Type IV	All other harmful procedures to the female genitalia for non-medical purposes, for example: pricking, piercing, incising, scraping and cauterization.

[1]Reprinted from World Health Organization. Eliminating female genital mutilation: an interagency statement UNAIDS, UNDP, UNECA, UNESCO, UNFPA, UNHCHR, UNHCR, UNICEF, UNIFEM, WHO. World Health Organization: Geneva. p. 24 (2008).

Appendix 6

Body mass index classifications

The International Classification of adult underweight, overweight and obesity according to BMI.

Classification	Body mass index (BMI–kg/m^2)
Underweight	< 18.50
Normal range	18.50–24.99
Overweight	25.00–29.99
Obese	> 30.00

Source: Reprinted from Body Mass Index–BMI. World Health Organization. 2017. Retrieved from: www.euro.who.int/en/health-topics/disease-prevention/nutrition/a-healthy-lifestyle/body-mass-index bmi